World of Cupping

World of Cupping

Cups of wellness- The Art of Hijama

Advanced Cupping Therapy: A Professional Guide to Modern Hijama Practices

By: Moe Ahmed

Copyright © 2024 by Moe Ahmed

The content contained within this book may not be reproduced, duplicated, or transmitted without direct written permission from the author or the publisher. Under no circumstances will any blame or legal responsibility be held against the publisher or author, for any damages, reparation, or monetary loss due to the information contained within the book, either directly or indirectly.

Legal Notice:

This book is copyright protected. It is only for personal use. You cannot amend, distribute, sell, use, quote, or paraphrase any part or the content within this book without the consent of the author or publisher.

Disclaimer Notice:

Please note the information contained within this document is for educational and entertainment purpose only. All effort has been executed to present accurate, up to date, reliable, complete information. No warranties of any kind are declared or implied. Readers acknowledge that the author is not engaged in the rendering of legal, financial, medical or professional advice. The content within this book has been derived from various sources. Please consult a licensed professional before attempting any techniques outlined in this book.

About the Author

Moe Ahmed is a passionate and experienced cupping therapy expert, who has dedicated his life to mastering and sharing the art of Hijama. Hijama, also known as cupping therapy, is a therapeutic practice that involves applying cups to specific points on the body to create suction and extract blood and fluids. It is based on the teachings and traditions of the Prophet Muhammad (SAW), who recommended it as a beneficial and effective treatment for various ailments.

Moe Ahmed learned Hijama from his father, who was a professional and skilled practitioner of this ancient technique. His father's career and passion inspired him to follow his footsteps and pursue Hijama as his own calling. He started practicing Hijama on his family members when he was 18 years old, and soon realized the immense potential and value of this healing method.

He decided to further his education and expertise in Hijama by studying at renowned institutions in the UK, California, and Turkey, where he gained exposure to different aspects and approaches of cupping therapy. He also acquired world-class certifications from IPHM, and joined prestigious associations such as the London Hijama Academy. He has been constantly updating his knowledge and skills in Hijama, as well as exploring other related fields such as sports therapy and Swedish American massage.

Moe Ahmed is not only a service provider, but also a global pioneer and leader in holistic wellness. He sees himself as a custodian of a tradition, but with a modern and innovative vision. He strives to offer an impeccable blend of time-tested practices and cutting-edge techniques to his clients, who range from ordinary people to elite athletes. He has worked with members of the USA cricket team, UFC fighters, and renowned basketball players, who have all benefited from his excellence and expertise in Hijama.

Moe Ahmed loves Hijama and considers it his passion and mission. He is always eager to learn more and teach others about this amazing art of healing. He hopes that his book, World of Cupping: Beyond the Blood - The Art of Hijama, will inspire and educate readers about the wonders and benefits of Hijama, and help them achieve holistic health and athletic excellence.

Table of Contents

Chapter
01

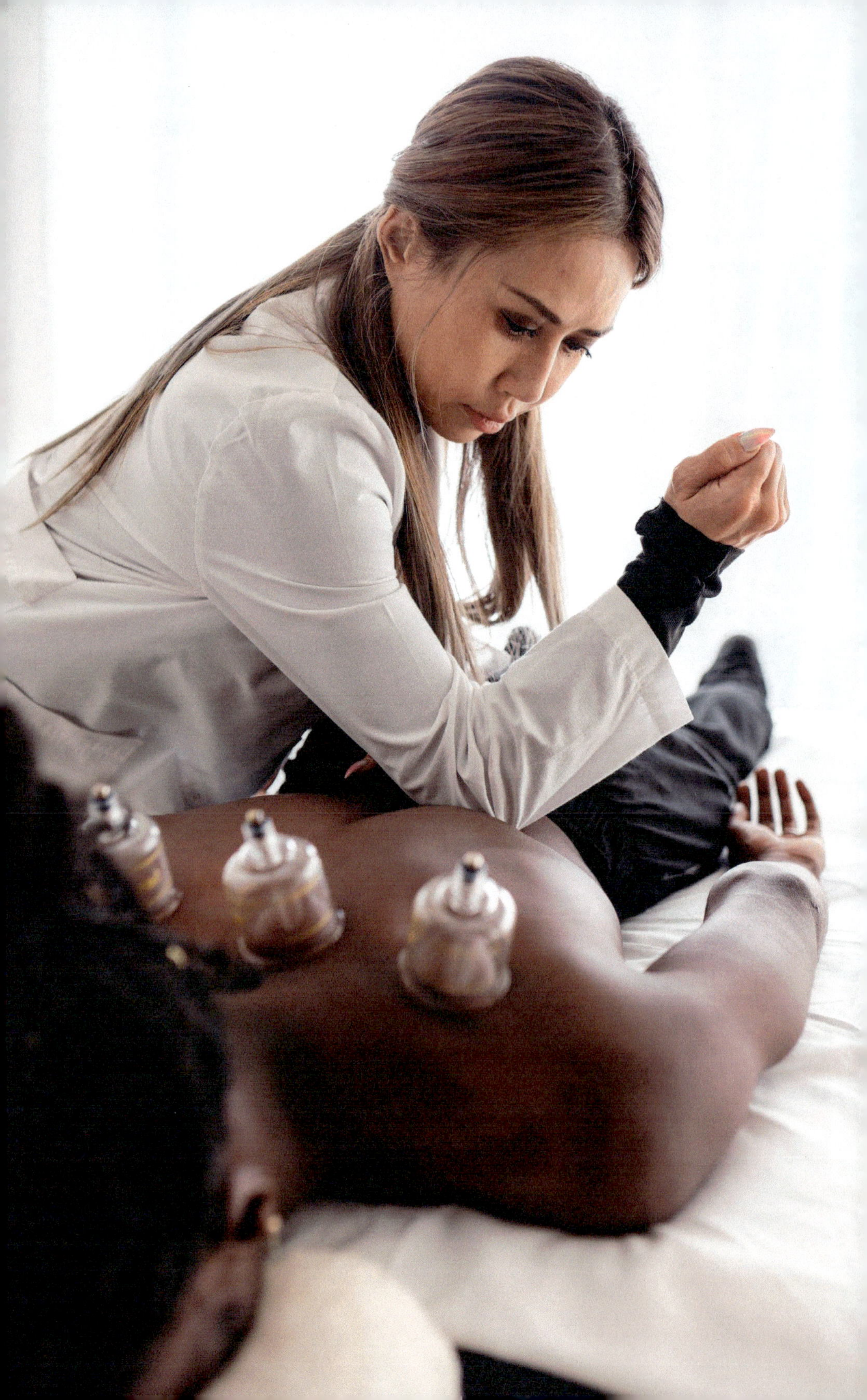

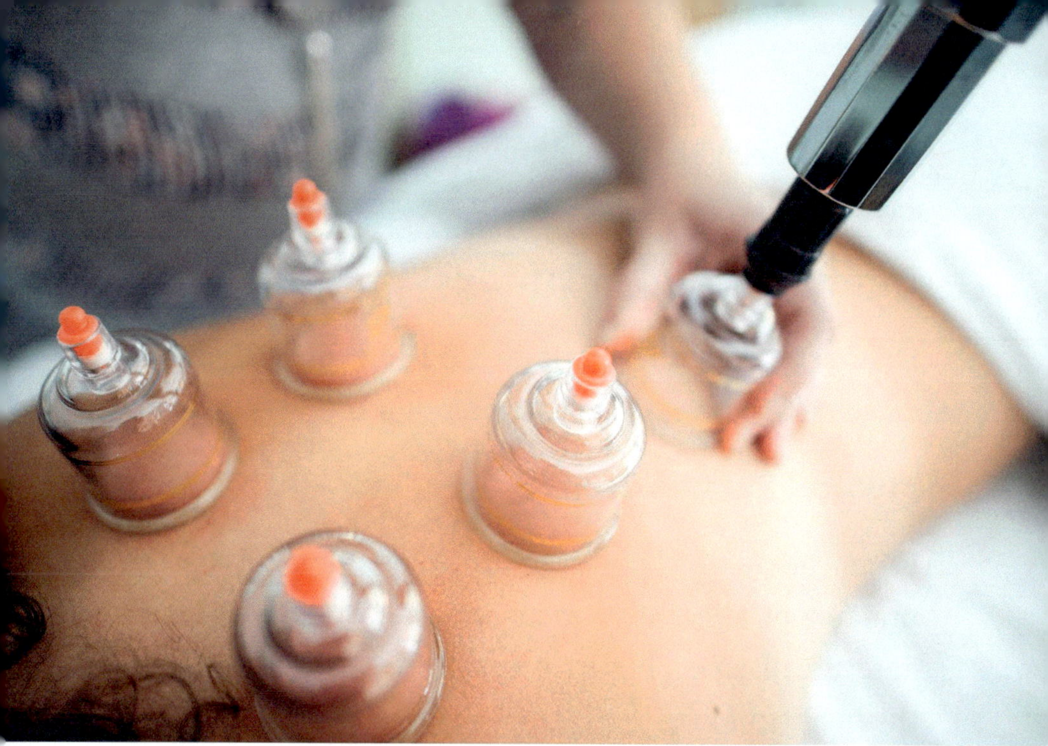

Introduction to Hijama cupping therapy

This chapter will explain what Hijama cupping therapy is, how it differs from other types of cupping, and why it is good to health and wellness. You will also learn about the history and evolution of Hijama cupping therapy, including the contributions of numerous civilizations and cultures, particularly Islam, to its growth.

Hijama cupping therapy is a holistic therapeutic technique that includes placing suction cups to particular locations on the body and extracting blood and toxins through tiny incisions. The word Hijama is derived from the Arabic root hajm, which means sucking. Hijama cupping therapy is often referred to as bloodletting, wet cupping, or blood cupping.

Definition and Meaning:

Hijama cupping therapy is defined and comprehended from three perspectives: medical, scientific, and spiritual.

Medical Perspective:

From the medical perception, Hijama cupping therapy is a practice of alternative medicine that objectives to prevent and cure diseases, improve health and wellness, and enhance the quality of life.

Hijama cupping therapy is founded on the ideas of traditional medicine, including Ayurveda (Indian) and Unani (Greco-Arabic), which see the human body as a complex system of interconnected parts, including tissues (structures), organs (functions), humors (fluids), and temperaments (personalities).

Hijama cupping treatment functions by eliminating excess or dangerous chemicals that lead to illness and dysfunction and by bringing these elements back into harmony and balance.

Scientific perspective:

According to science, Hijama cupping treatment is a type of biomedical engineering that modifies the human body and its processes by using the laws of physics, chemistry, and biology. Hijama cupping therapy functions by applying a negative pressure to the skin, which widens the blood vessels, increases blood flow, activates the lymphatic system, stimulates the nervous system, and releases endorphins, which are the body's natural analgesics. Another way that Hijama cupping therapy functions is by causing a controlled bleeding, which leads to blood coagulation (clotting), waste product removal, blood viscosity (thickness) reduction, blood cell regeneration, and immune system stimulation.

Spiritual Perspective:

From a spiritual standpoint, Hijama cupping treatment is a type of divine healing that adheres to the principles and practices of Islam, the faith revealed by Allah (God) to the Prophet Muhammad (peace be upon him) in the seventh century CE. Hijama cupping therapy is not only a medical treatment, but also a religious obligation and a form of devotion for Muslims, as it is based on the Prophet Muhammad's (peace be upon him) Sunnah. Hijama cupping treatment connects the body and spirit while also improving self-awareness and attention towards the Creator. Hijama cupping treatment also works by regulating the flow of life energy (qi in Chinese medicine, prana in Ayurveda, or ruh in Islam) and balancing the yin and yang energies in the body.

Hijama in the Light of Ahaadeeth

Hijama is a therapeutic technique that includes placing cups in particular places on the body to generate suction and collect blood and fluids. It is based on the Prophet Muhammad's

(SAW) teachings and traditions, which endorsed it as a useful and effective cure for a variety of diseases. His distinguished associates (RA) documented his Hijama-related sayings and acts in the Ahaadeeth volumes, which serve us with important advice and insight on the subject. In this section, I will concentrate on the Ahaadeeth that highlight the advantages and benefits of Hijama, as well as those that suggest the permissibility of collecting a price for the service. The Ahaadeeth about the cost are significant because some people believe that Hijama should be performed for free, which violates the Prophet's Sunnah. Other Ahaadeeth that deal with the specific aspects and facts of Hijama will be discussed in their respective chapters.

The Virtues and Benefits of Hijama

Hijama is a highly praised and recommended practice in Islam, as evident from the following Ahaadeeth:

1. **Jabir bin Abdullaah (RA) reported** that he heard the Prophet (SAW) saying: "The best of your remedies is hijama. It removes blood, lightens the back and sharpens the eyesight." (Bukhari and Muslim)

2. **Asim b. 'Umar b. Qatada (RA) narrated**: 'Abdullaah and another person from his household came to our house complaining of a wound. Jabir (RA) asked: What is wrong with you? He said: I have a wound that is very painful. Jabir (RA) said: Boy, bring me a cupper. He

said: 'Abdullaah, what do you want to do with the cupper? I said: I want to have this wound cupped. He said: By Allaah, even the touch of a fly or a cloth hurts me (and cupping) would cause me unbearable pain. When he saw him suffering (from the idea of cupping), he said: I heard the Messenger of Allaah (SAW) saying: The most effective of your treatments are hijama, honey, and cauterization with fire, but I do not like to be cauterized. The cupper was brought and he cupped him and he was cured. (Sahih Muslim 26:5468)

3. **Abu Hurayrah (RA) related that** Abu Hind (RA) cupped the Prophet (SAW) on the center of his head. The Prophet (SAW) said: O Banu Bayadah, marry Abu Hind (to your daughter), and ask him to marry (his daughter) to you. He said: The best thing that you use for healing is hijama. (Abu Dawud 5:2097)

4. **Abu Hurayrah (RA) reported** that the Prophet (SAW) said: The best treatment that you use is hijama. (Abu Dawud 22:3848)

5. **Abu Hurayrah (RA) narrated** that the Prophet (SAW) said: "Whoever performs hijama on the 17th, 19th or 21st of the month, it will be a cure for him from every disease." (Sahih Al-Jaami' 5968)

6. **Abu Hurayrah (RA) narrated** that the Prophet (SAW) said: "Jibra'eel came to me and said: O Muhammad,

order your Ummah to do hijama, for it is the best of what they use for healing." (Sahih Al-Jaami 213)

7. **Abdullaah ibn Abbas (RA) reported** that the Prophet (SAW) said, "I did not pass by any angel on the night of ascension except that they all said to me: You should do hijama, O Muhammad." [Saheeh Sunan ibn Maajah (3477).

8. In the narration reported by Abdullaah ibn Mas'ud (RA) the angels said, "Oh Muhammad, order your Ummah (nation) with Hijamah." [Saheeh Sunan Tirmidhi (3479)]

9. **Rasulullaah (Sallallaahu Álayhi Wasallam)** said, 'Jibraaeel (Álayhis salaam) repeatedly emphasized upon me to resort to Hijamah to the extent that I feared that Hijamah will be made compulsory.' (Jamúl Wasaail p. 179).

10. **Rasulullaah (Sallallaahu Álayhi Wasallam)** praised a person who performs Hijamah, saying it removes blood, lightens the back and sharpens the eyesight (Jamúl Wasaail p. 179)

11. **Hadhrat Abu Kabsha (Radhiallaahu Ánhu)** narrates that Rasulullaah (Sallallaahu Álayhi Wasallam) used to undergo cupping on the head and between his shoulders and he used to say, 'Whosoever removes this blood, it will not harm him that he does not take any other medical treatment.' (Mishkāt p. 389).

Hijama vs Donating Blood

Hijama and blood donation are two separate procedures that entail extracting blood from the body, but they serve distinct objectives, techniques, and outcomes. Hijama is a medicinal technique that seeks to cleanse the body of toxins and impurities, whereas blood donation is a humanitarian gesture intended to save the lives of people who require blood transfusions. Hijama and donating blood vary in the following ways:

Source and Type of Blood

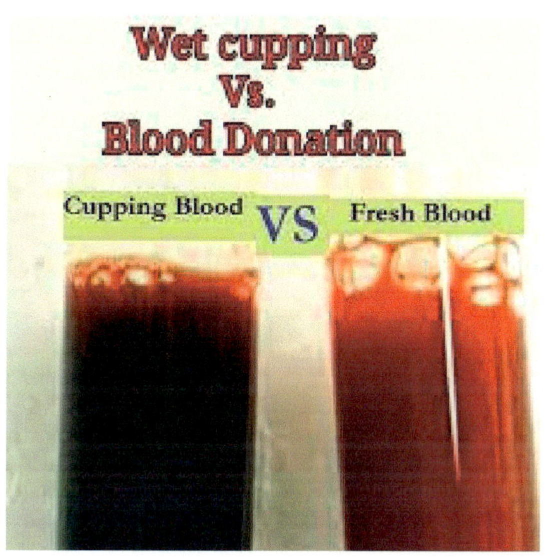

Hijama extract blood from the interstitial fluids, which are fluids between cells, and the capillaries, which are tiny blood arteries. Toxins and pollutants gather in these areas, and the Hijama aids in filtering and eliminating them. Typically, Hijama blood is thick, black, and odorous, which denotes its low quality and potential danger.

When someone donates blood, blood is used from the veins—the big blood arteries that return blood to the heart. Patients who have had operations, illnesses, or injuries can utilize this fresh, oxygenated, and healthy blood to replace the blood they have lost. Blood that has been donated is often thin, colorless, and brilliant red, suggesting that it is high-quality and beneficial.

Amount and Frequency of Blood

Hijama draws a small amount of blood, usually around 50 ml, from the surface of the skin. This blood is not essential for the body, and it can be easily replenished. Hijama can be done regularly, depending on the individual's condition and needs. The Prophet (SAW) recommended doing Hijama on certain days of the lunar month, such as the 17th, 19th, or 21st.

Donating blood takes a considerable volume of blood from the veins, often approximately 500 ml. This blood is essential to the body, and it takes time to replenish. Depending on the individual's health and eligibility, blood donation is only possible on occasion. Men should donate blood at least every 8 weeks, and women every 12 weeks.

Benefits and Risks of Blood

Hijama has several health advantages, including improved blood circulation, immune system stimulation, pain and

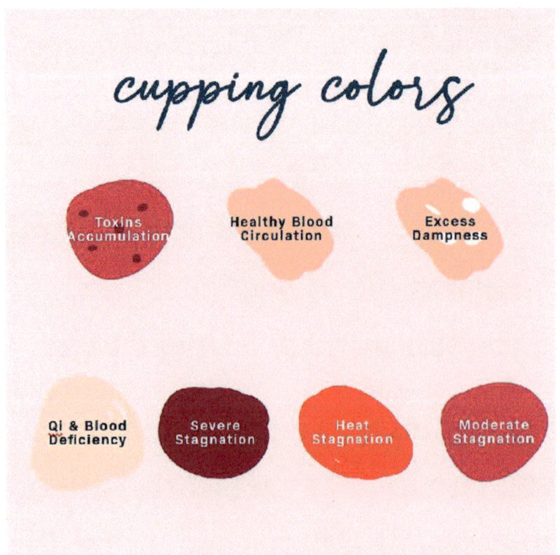

inflammation relief, and illness treatment. Hijama also offers spiritual advantages, such as reversing the effects of the evil eye, sorcery, and jinn possession. Hijama has limited dangers, such as bruising, swelling, or infection, which may be avoided by practicing adequate cleanliness and measures.

Donating blood provides certain benefits for the donor, including decreased blood pressure, cholesterol, and improved mood. Donating blood offers several advantages for the recipient, including saving lives, enhancing health, and restoring blood volume. Donating blood carries various dangers, including fainting, hemorrhage, and iron shortage, which may be prevented by adhering to adequate rules and care.

The ancient origins and practices of Hijama cupping therapy

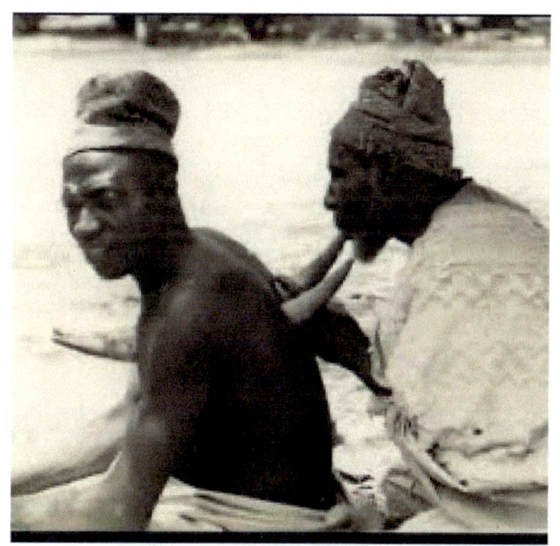

Hijama cupping medical therapy is one of the oldest and most widely used therapeutic procedures in human history. It has been performed by civilizations and cultures all throughout the world, from antiquity to the present. The following are some historical milestones and advancements in Hijama cupping therapy:

Egypt

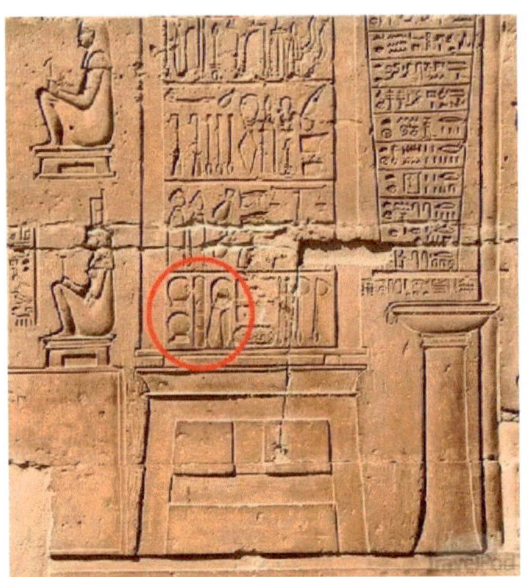

Hijama cupping therapy was used in ancient Egypt, as demonstrated by the Ebers Papyrus, the earliest medical record dating back to 1550 BC and mentioning the use of cupping for numerous diseases. The Ebers Papyrus contains almost 700 formulae and cures for a wide range of ailments and disorders, including headaches, stomachaches, skin issues, vision difficulties, and snake stings. The Ebers Papyrus also covers the many forms and procedures of cupping, such as wet cupping, dry cupping, and moving cupping, as well as the places and indications of cupping, which include the back, neck, shoulders, and legs. The Ebers Papyrus also cites the use of animal horns, clay pots, and glass containers as cupping tools. The ancient Egyptians thought that cupping could balance the body's four humors (blood, phlegm, yellow bile, and black bile) and remove bad spirits and negative energies that caused sickness and disorder.

China

Hijama cupping treatment was employed in ancient China, as demonstrated by the Huangdi Neijing, the earliest medical treatise dating back to 300 BC and mentioning the use of cupping for numerous ailments. The Huangdi Neijing, commonly known as the Yellow Emperor's Classic of Internal Medicine, is Chinese medicine's core work, including the ideas and concepts of anatomy, physiology, pathology, diagnosis, therapy, and illness prevention. The Huangdi Neijing also details the many forms and procedures of cupping, including

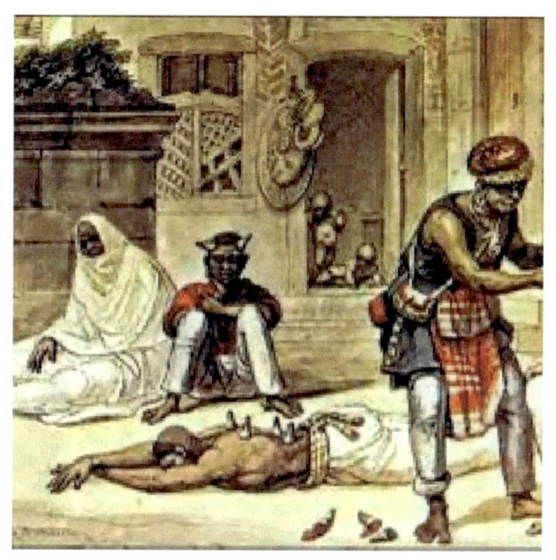

wet cupping, dry cupping, fire cupping, and bamboo cupping, as well as the places and indications of cupping, which include the back, chest, belly, and limbs. The Huangdi Neijing also includes animal horns, bamboo tubes, ceramic jars, and metal pots as cupping devices. The ancient Chinese thought that cupping could control the flow of qi (life energy) and blood in the body, as well as balance the yin and yang (opposite and complementary energies).

Greece and Rome

Hijama cupping treatment was performed in ancient Greece and Rome, as proven by the works of Hippocrates, the founder of medicine, and Galen, the prince of physicians, both of

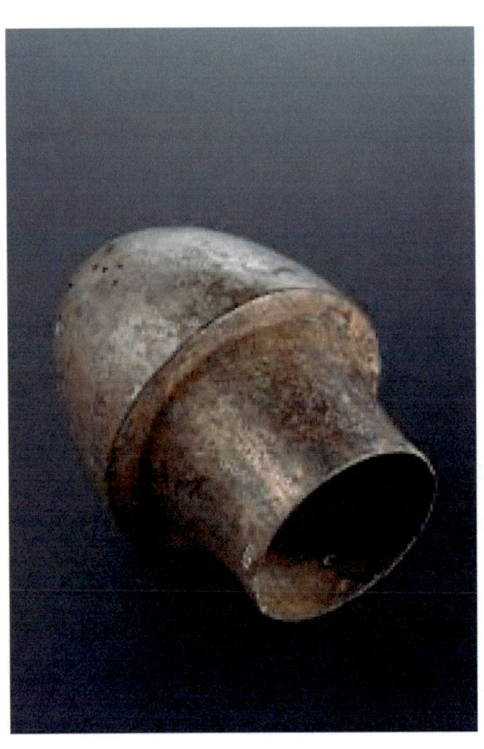

whom recommended cupping for a variety of conditions. Hippocrates, who lived in the fifth and fourth century BC, created the Hippocratic Corpus, a collection of over 60 medical treatises on anatomy, physiology, pathology, diagnosis, therapy, and illness prevention. Hippocrates also produced the Aphorisms, a compilation of over 400 succinct and useful remarks summarizing medical concepts and guidelines. Hippocrates also created the Oath, a physician-specific rule of ethics and conduct that is still in use today. Hippocrates also outlined the several types and procedures of cupping, such as wet cupping, dry cupping, and moving cupping, as well as the places and reasons for cupping, which included the head, neck, chest, and joints. Hippocrates also suggested the use of animal horns, metal cups, and glass cups for cupping. Hippocrates also thought that cupping could balance the body's four humors (blood, phlegm, yellow bile, and black bile) and eliminate excess or poisonous substances that caused sickness and disorder.

Galen, who lived in the second and third century AD, produced nearly 500 medical volumes on themes such as anatomy, physiology, pathology, diagnosis, therapy, and illness prevention. Galen also composed the Commentaries, a collection of commentaries and explanations of Hippocrates' 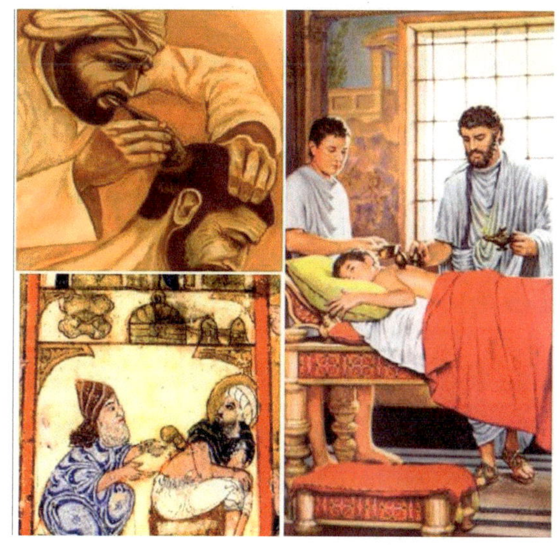 writings, which he respected and emulated. Galen also authored On the Therapeutic Method, a treatise about the ideas and practices of medical therapy, which he classified into three categories: food, medicines, and surgery. Galen also discussed the many types and methods of cupping, including as wet cupping, dry cupping, and fire cupping, as well as the places and indications for cupping, which included the back, chest, belly, and limbs. Galen also referenced the use of animal horns, metal cups, and glass cups as cupping tools. Galen also thought that cupping could control the flow of pneuma (breath or spirit) and blood in the body, as well as balance the temperaments (personalities) and complexions (colors).

The Art and Science of Hijama: A Detailed Exploration

Hijama, also known as cupping treatment, is an ancient procedure that includes placing suction cups on the skin to improve blood flow and eliminate impurities. Hijama practitioners must have a thorough understanding of numerous elements of health and healing, including:

Temperaments:

The four humors or bodily fluids that influence the physical and mental characteristics of a person. They are blood, phlegm, yellow bile, and black bile. Hijama practitioners need to assess the balance of these humors in each patient and adjust the treatment accordingly.

Acupuncture:

A form of alternative medicine that involves inserting thin needles into specific points on the body to regulate the flow of qi (vital energy) and restore health. Hijama practitioners may use acupuncture points as reference for locating the Hijama points and enhancing the effects of cupping.

Phytotherapy:

The use of plant-based medicines to treat various diseases and conditions. Hijama practitioners may use herbs, oils, or extracts to prepare the skin before cupping, to apply on the cupped areas after removing the cups, or to give as oral or topical remedies to the patients.

Reflexology:

A type of massage that involves applying pressure to specific areas on the feet, hands, or ears that correspond to different organs and body systems. Hijama practitioners may use reflexology to diagnose and treat the patients, as well as to complement the cupping therapy.

Naturopathy:

A system of health care that promotes the body's own self-healing ability and uses natural therapies such as nutrition, exercise, and stress management. Hijama practitioners may use naturopathy to educate and advise the patients on how to prevent and treat diseases holistically and naturally.

Diagnosis of Diseases by Traditional Methods

The use of diverse procedures and instruments to detect illness causes and symptoms through observation, history, examination, and intuition. Hijama practitioners may employ pulse diagnosis, tongue diagnosis, urine analysis, or facial diagnosis to identify the optimal treatment approach for each patient.

What You Need to Know About When to Do Hijama?

Hijama frequency depends on several factors, such as:

The health condition of the patient:

Hijama could help with a variety of conditions and symptoms, including pain, inflammation, infection, blood pressure, diabetes, and more. The frequency with which Hijama should be worn may vary according on the severity and kind of ailment. For example, chronic diseases may need more frequent treatments than acute ones.

The lunar calendar and the Sunnah days:

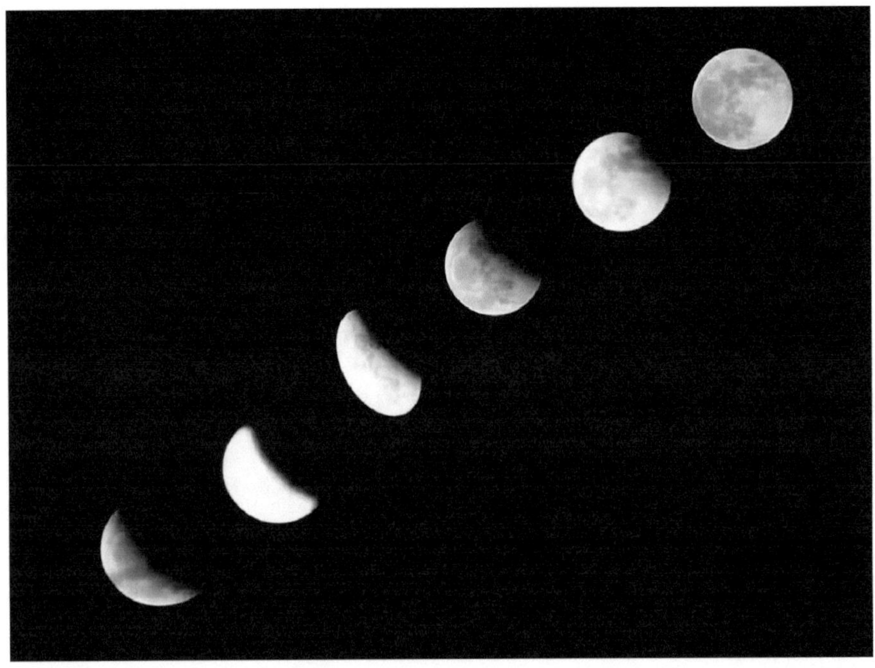

Hijama is governed by lunar phases, therefore certain days are more fortunate and helpful than others. The Prophet Muhammad (peace be upon him) suggested that the 17th, 19th, and 21st of the lunar month be the finest days for Hijama.

The individual preference and the tolerance of the patient:

Hijama may be modified and changed to meet the patient's demands and comfort. Some patients may prefer more or less sessions, cups, suction, and so on. The Hijama practitioner should honor the patient's preferences and input and adjust the therapy accordingly.

What is screening cupping therapy?

It is a cupping therapy that takes four sessions and treats the body as a whole. As a result of the four sessions, the entire body is cleaned and the immune system strengthened. The treatment has a significant and long-term influence.

The preventative or therapeutic effect on ailments is stronger. This is because a sickness in one part of the body may impact the whole body.

Skin disorders, migraines, muscle and joint problems, chronic diseases including diabetes, psychological ailments, and Alzheimer's disease are all excellent candidates for screening cupping therapy.

How Hijama Cupping Therapy Is Different from Other Forms of Cupping?

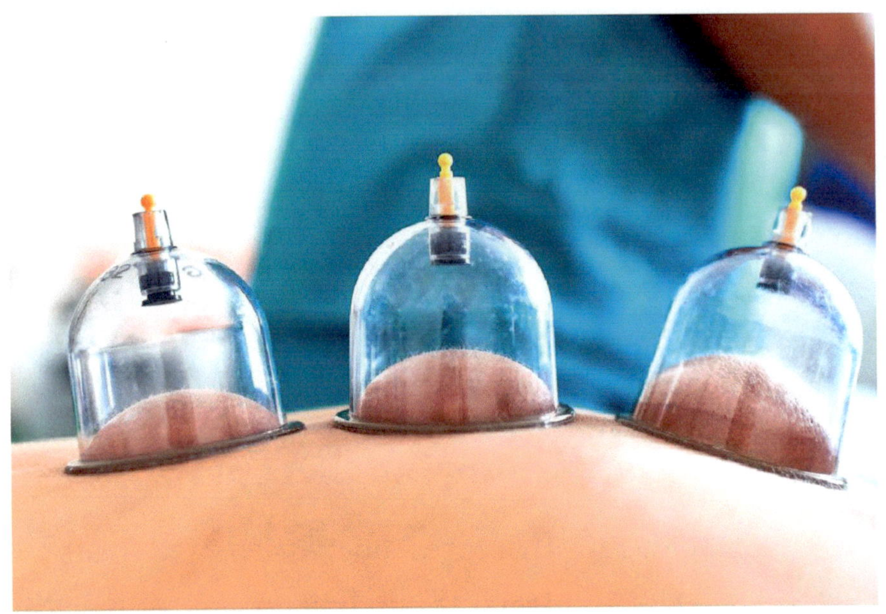

Hijama cupping treatment differs from other types of cupping, such as dry cupping and fire cupping, which do not include bloodletting. Dry cupping and fire cupping simply create a vacuum on the skin by lifting and stimulating blood flow with air or heat. Hijama cupping therapy, on the other hand, entails cutting small wounds in the skin before applying the cups to collect blood and impurities from the body.

The primary distinction between Hijama cupping therapy and other types of cupping is the goal and result of the suction. The objective of suction in dry cupping and fire cupping is to enhance blood flow to the afflicted region, while the impact is to widen the blood vessels and relax the muscles. The goal of Hijama cupping therapy is to reduce blood flow to the afflicted area, and the suction has the effect of constricting blood vessels and contracting muscles.

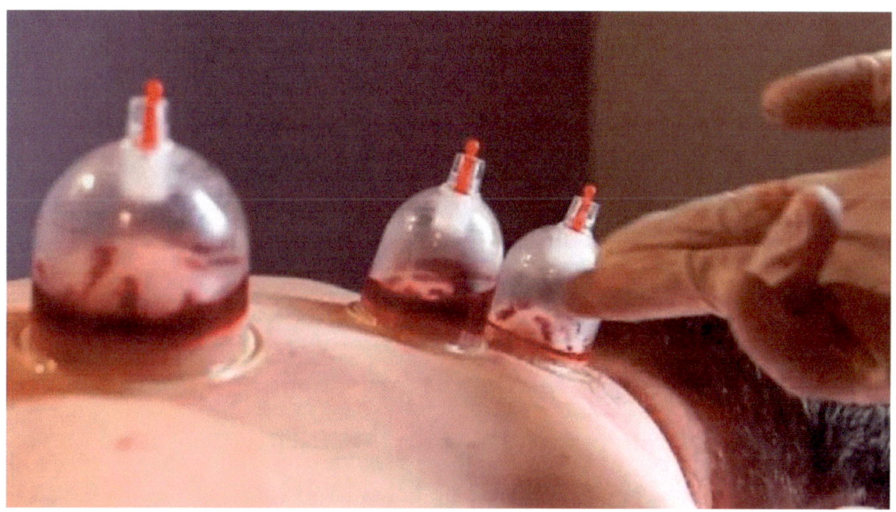

This discrepancy is due to the presence or lack of incisions. There are no incisions made on the skin during dry cupping or fire cupping, so the blood stays inside the body and circulates naturally. In Hijama cupping therapy, incisions are created in the skin, allowing blood to seep out of the body and gather inside the cups.

The advantage of this variation is the elimination or retention of blood and poisons. Dry and fire cupping hold blood and toxins inside the body, which can lead to inflammation, illness, or stagnation. Hijama cupping treatment removes blood and toxins from the body, which may help in pain relief, wound healing, and blood purification.

Hijama Aftermath: Unraveling Possible Reactions

Hijama is generally a safe and well-tolerated procedure, but it may have some side effects or complications, such as:

Bruising, swelling, or pain at the cupping sites:

These are the most common and minor adverse effects of Hijama, and they normally go away within a few days. They can be mitigated by administering cold, compression, or topical treatments to the afflicted regions. Furthermore, putting olive oil or black sesame oil on the skin helps decrease inflammation and aid healing. Olive and black seed oil are natural oils with anti-inflammatory, antibacterial, and antioxidant effects. They can also keep the skin moisturized and scar-free. To use, use a few drops of oil on the bruised or swollen region and gently massage until absorbed. Repeat twice a day until the symptoms have subsided.

Infection, bleeding, or scarring at the cupping sites:

These are uncommon yet significant consequences of Hijama, particularly if wet or hot cupping is employed. They may be avoided by utilizing sterile equipment, maintaining good cleanliness, and providing adequate wound care.

Anemia, dehydration, or fatigue:

These are potential side effects of Hijama, especially if large amounts of blood are removed or if Hijama is done too frequently or for too long. They can be avoided by drinking plenty of fluids, eating nutritious foods, and resting after the procedure.

Allergic reactions, drug interactions, or contraindications:

These are some of the probable negative effects of Hijama, particularly if herbs, oils, or other substances are used during or following the operation. They can be avoided by reviewing the patient's medical history, allergies, medicines, and health status prior to applying Hijama.

Academic Studies Examining the Efficacy of Hijama:

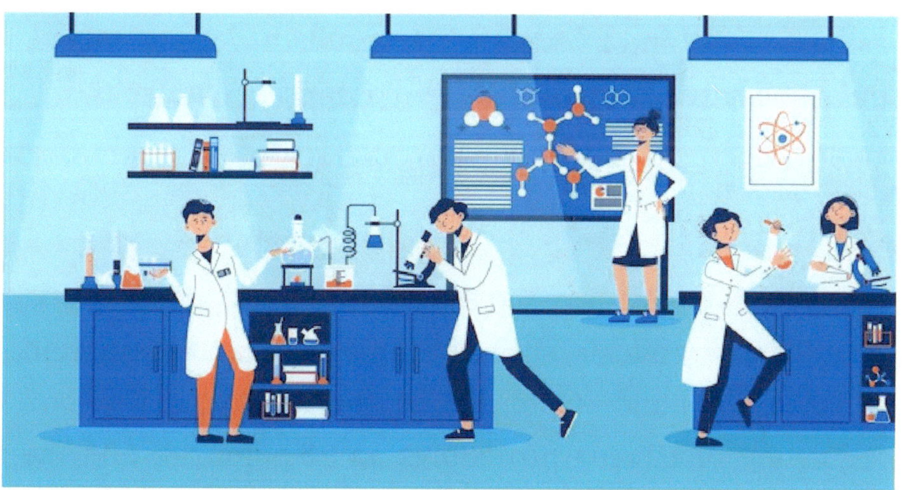

Hijama is an ancient and traditional practice that has been gaining more attention and interest from the scientific and medical community in recent years. There are many academic researches about Hijama, such as:

The effects of Hijama on pain, inflammation, immune system, blood circulation, and oxidative stress:

Many studies have shown that Hijama can reduce pain, inflammation, and oxidative stress, and improve immune system function and blood circulation, by modulating various biochemical and physiological mechanisms.

The efficacy of Hijama for various diseases and conditions:

Many studies have evaluated the efficacy of Hijama for various diseases and conditions, such as hypertension, diabetes, migraine, low back pain, rheumatoid arthritis, asthma, acne, and infertility. The results have been mixed, but some have shown positive and promising outcomes.

The safety and quality of Hijama practice and products:

Many studies have assessed the safety and quality of Hijama practice and products, such as the incidence and prevention of side effects and complications, the standardization and regulation of Hijama procedures and equipment, and the quality and analysis of Hijama blood and cupping marks.

The findings have highlighted the need for more guidelines, training, and monitoring of Hijama practice and products.

Benefits Hijama cupping:

Hijama cupping therapy provides several physical, mental, emotional, and spiritual advantages. Some of the advantages and consequences of Hijama cupping therapy include:

Physical Level

On a physical level, Hijama cupping therapy cleanses and purifies the blood while also improving blood circulation. It eliminates toxic toxins and infections from the body and strengthens the immune system. It controls hormone homeostasis as well as organ and gland function. It reduces pain and inflammation while healing injuries and wounds. It lowers the chance of acquiring chronic and degenerative diseases such diabetes, hypertension, heart disease, cancer, and Alzheimer's disease.

Mental Level

Hijama cupping treatment helps to alleviate tension and anxiety while also promoting relaxation and well-being. It increases cognitive skills like memory, attention, focus, and learning. It improves mood and emotional stability while also preventing or treating mental diseases including depression, sleeplessness, and schizophrenia.

Emotional Level

Hijama cupping treatment helps eliminate bad emotions and traumas from the body and subconscious mind. It assists in overcoming psychological and emotional disorders such as wrath, fear, guilt, humiliation, and resentment. It promotes pleasant feelings and attitudes, like love, appreciation, forgiveness, and compassion. It enhances interpersonal interactions and social skills while also boosting self-esteem and confidence levels.

Spiritual Level

Hijama cupping therapy enhances the spiritual link between the body and soul, increasing self-awareness and mindfulness towards the Creator. It cleanses the heart and spirit of sins and ills, increasing faith and piety. It harmonizes the body and spirit with natural laws and divine will, increasing blessings and rewards in this life and the hereafter.

Chapter 02

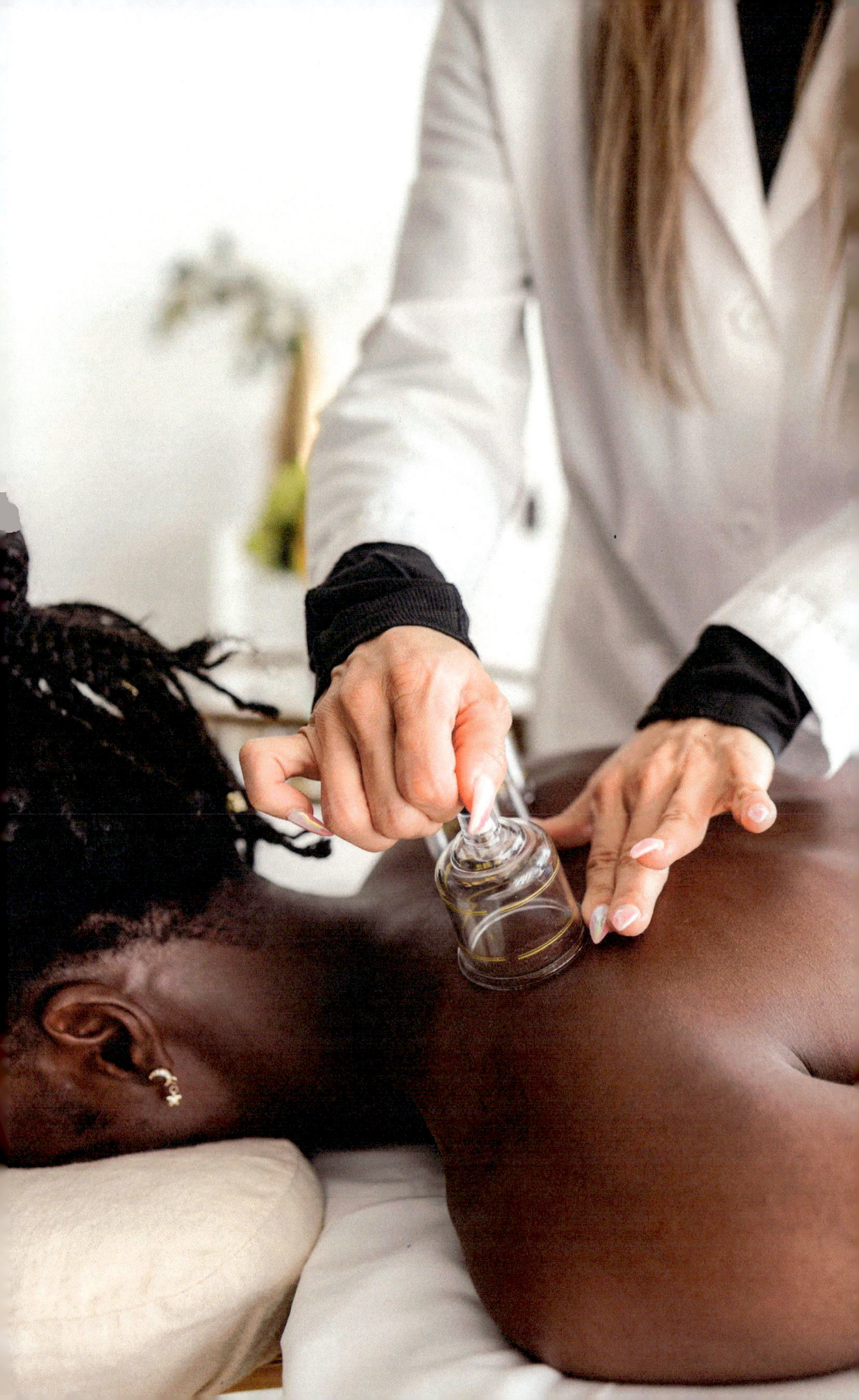

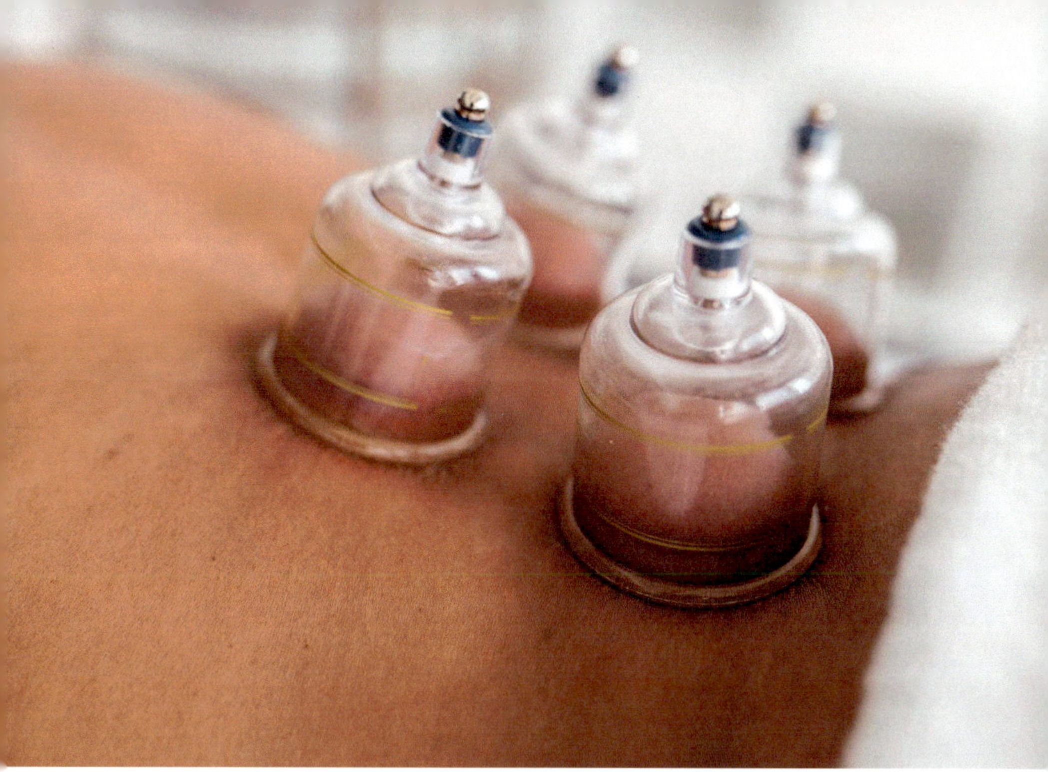

How Did Hijama Cupping Therapy Originate and Develop Over Time?

This chapter will teach you about the history and progress of Hijama cupping therapy, from ancient times to the present. You will also learn about how numerous civilizations and cultures, including Egypt, China, Greece, Rome, Africa, Arabia, Europe, and America, contributed to the growth of Hijama cupping therapy. Hijama cupping treatment is an alternative medical technique that includes producing suction on the skin with cups to promote blood flow, eliminate toxins, and balance the body's energy. Hijama cupping treatment has been used for thousands of years by people across the world for a variety of objectives, including healing, preventive, and spiritual improvement.

The Ancient Legacy of Hijama: A 50,000-Year Therapeutic Tradition

Hijama has a very old history, dating back to ancient civilizations including Egypt, China, and the Middle East.

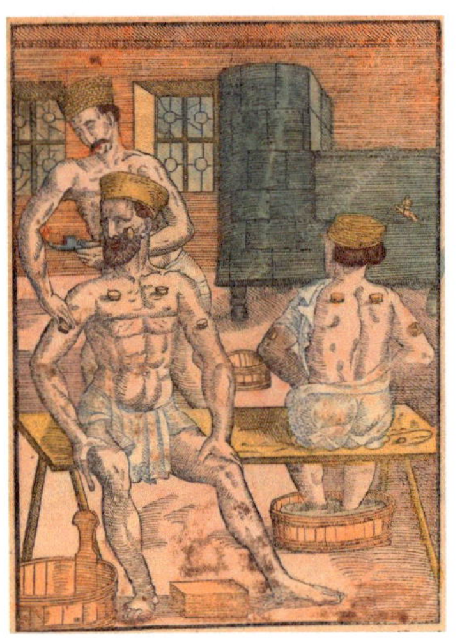

Some reports indicate that the ancient Egyptians performed Hijama as early as 50,000 years ago, using animal horns as cups.

Hijama Across Continents: A Historical Journey from Egypt and Asia to Anatolia and Europe

Hijama was performed by many nations and areas, including China, India, Persia, Greece, Rome, and Africa, in addition to ancient Egypt. Hijama traveled from Egypt and Asia to Anatolia and Europe via commerce, migration, and conquest. Hijama was inspired and shaped by other cultures' medical traditions and beliefs, including Ayurveda, Hippocratic medicine, and Islamic medicine. Hijama became a component of the religious and cultural practices of many faiths, including Judaism, Christianity, and Islam.

Hijama in China

Silk Road traders and travelers introduced Hijama to China, bringing with them expertise and methods from the Middle East and Central Asia. Hijama was included into Chinese medicine, which is founded on the notion of qi (vital energy) and the balance of yin and yang (opposite forces). Hijama was used to regulate the flow of qi and blood and to cure a variety of ailments, including colds, fevers, headaches, and arthritis. Hijama was also related with Taoism and acupuncture.

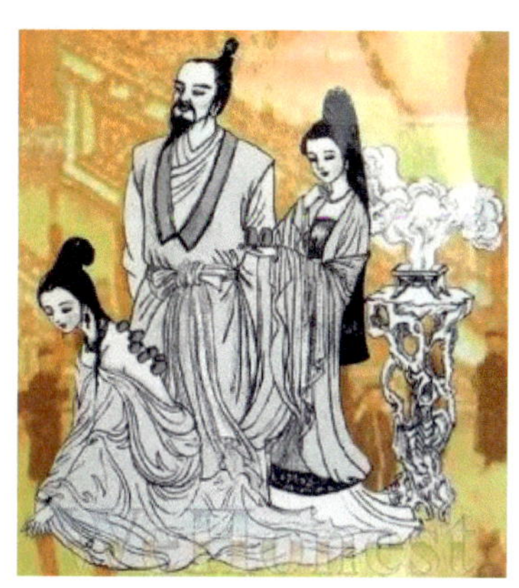

Hijama in India

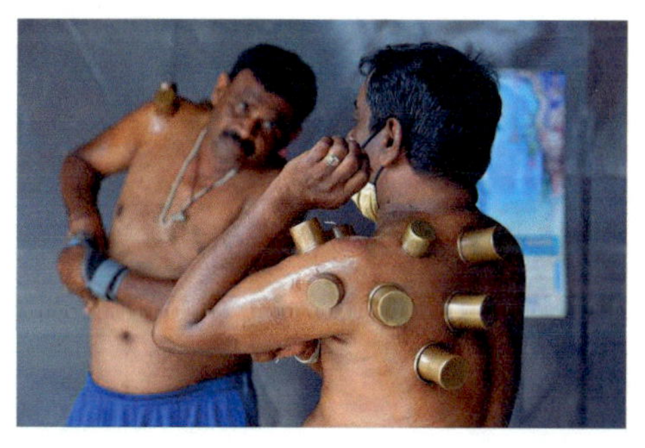

The ancient Hindus of India practiced Hijama, which they referred to as vedh or vedha. Hijama was a component of Ayurvedic treatment, which is founded on the notion of dosha (body type) and the balance of vata, pitta, and kapha (elements). Hijama was used to balance the dosha and heal a variety of ailments, including skin disorders, digestive troubles, and respiratory infections. Hijama was also impacted by Buddhist and Jain traditions, followed by Islamic and British influences.

Hijama in Europe

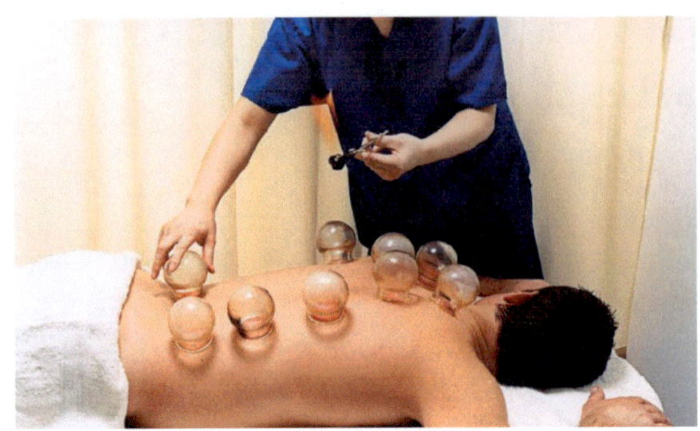

Greek and Roman physicians brought Hijama to Europe after learning it from Egyptians and Persians. Hijama was part of Hippocratic medicine, which was founded on the notion of humors (bodily fluids) and the balance of blood, phlegm, yellow bile, and black bile. Hijama was used to balance the humors and cure a variety of conditions, including gout, rheumatism, and epilepsy. Hijama was influenced by Christian and Jewish traditions, followed by Islamic and Renaissance influences.

Where did Hijama cupping therapy originate?

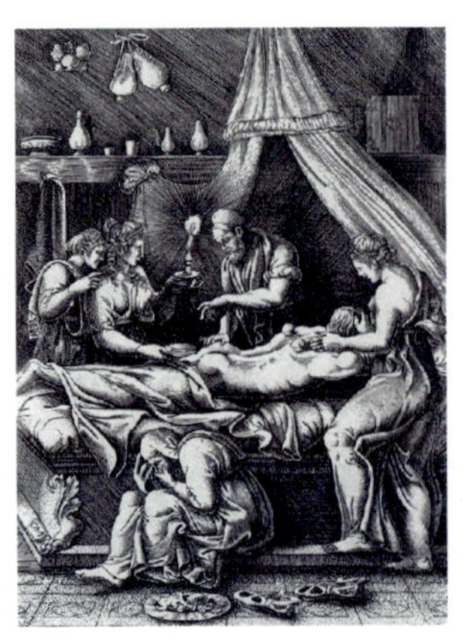

Hijama cupping treatment is one of the oldest and most widely used therapeutic procedures in human history. It has been performed by civilizations and cultures all throughout the world, from antiquity to the present. The following are some historical milestones and advancements in Hijama cupping therapy:

Ancient Origins

The history and practice of Hijama cupping treatment in Egypt, China, Greece, Rome, Africa, and Arabia. Hijama cupping treatment dates back over 5000 years, when it was utilized by the ancient Egyptians, Chinese, Greeks, Romans, Africans, and Arabs to heal a variety of ailments, injuries, illnesses, poisons, and curses. Hijama cupping therapy was also regarded as a holy and spiritual activity, since it was thought to purge bad spirits and negative energy from the body and psyche. Hijama cupping therapy was mentioned in

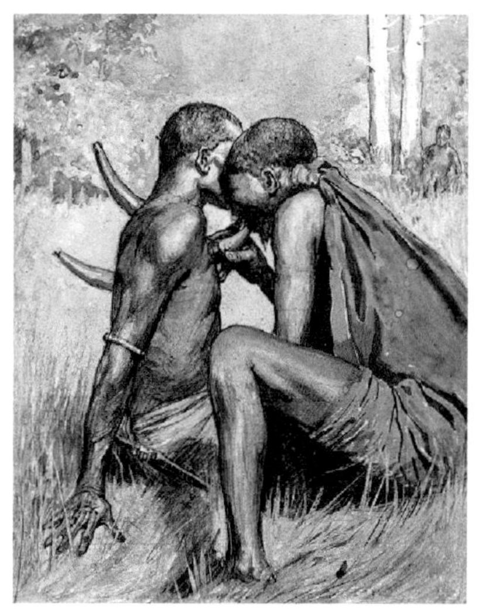

many ancient texts and scriptures, such as the Ebers Papyrus (the oldest medical document from Egypt), the Huangdi Neijing (the foundational text of Chinese medicine), the Hippocratic Corpus (the collection of writings by the father of Western medicine), the Kitab al-Tasrif (the influential medical encyclopedia by the Arab physician Al-Zahrawi), and the Canon of Medicine.

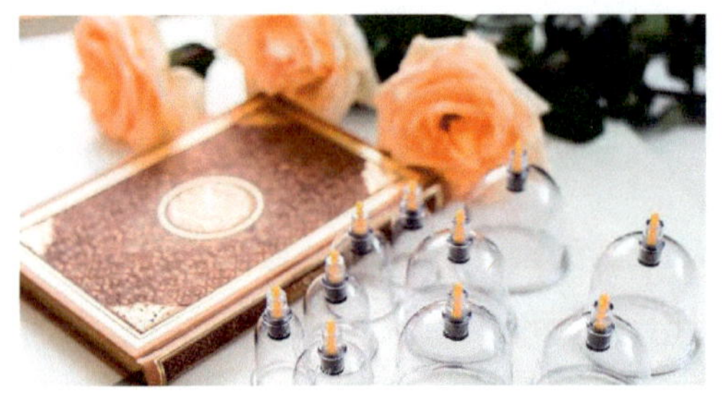

Islamic Perspective

The Islamic perspective and principles of Hijama cupping therapy, as well as its relevance in the Prophet Muhammad's Sunnah (peace be upon him). Hijama cupping therapy attained its pinnacle of popularity and excellence under the leadership and practice of Islam, the faith revealed by Allah (God) to the Prophet Muhammad (peace be upon him) in the seventh century CE. Hijama cupping therapy is not only a medical treatment, but also a religious obligation and a form of devotion for Muslims, as it is based on the Prophet Muhammad's (peace be upon him) Sunnah.

The Prophet Muhammad (peace be upon him) himself performed and recommended Hijama cupping therapy for himself and his companions, and praised its benefits and virtues. He said: "The best of remedies is Hijama cupping therapy" (Bukhari and Muslim), and "If there is any good in your medical treatments, it is in the blade of the cupper, drinking honey, or cauterization with fire, as appropriate to the cause of the illness, but I would not like to be cauterized" (Bukhari). He also said: "Whoever performs Hijama cupping therapy on the 17th, 19th, or 21st day (of the Islamic lunar calendar), then it is a cure for every disease" (Abu Dawud and Ibn Majah). He also described the optimal times, places, and procedures for administering Hijama cupping treatment, as well as cautioned against its overuse and abuse.

Historical Development

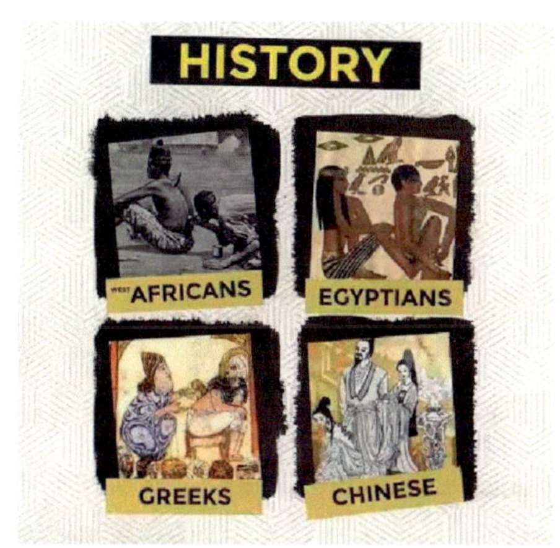

Historical development and spread of Hijama cupping therapy throughout Europe, America, and the rest of the world. Hijama cupping therapy moved from the Islamic world to Europe, America, and other parts of the world via commerce, travel, and cultural interchange. Hijama cupping therapy has been adopted and developed by many medical systems and schools, including the Unani (Greco-Arabic), Ayurvedic (Indian), Tibetan, Native American, and Western. Hijama cupping treatment was used to cure a variety of ailments, including fever, headache, cold, cough, asthma, arthritis, gout, sciatica, back pain, menstruation issues, digestive disorders, nerve disorders, and mental diseases. Many prominent and powerful persons have used hijama cupping treatment, including the Greek philosopher Socrates, the Roman emperor Julius Caesar, the French monarch Louis XIV, the British prime minister Winston Churchill, and the American president Abraham Lincoln.

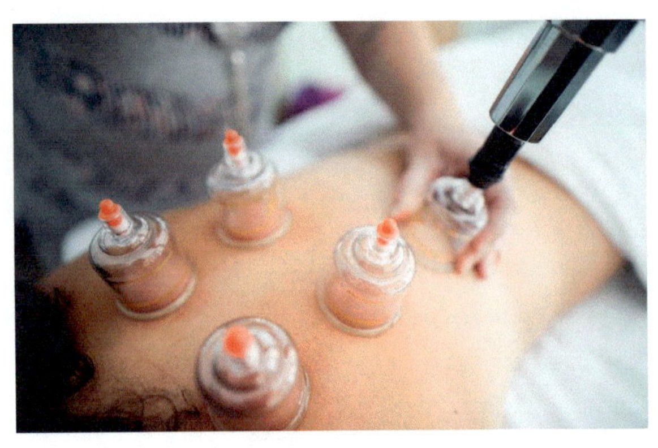

Modern Revival

Hijama cupping treatment is seeing a renaissance and growing appeal among Muslims and non-Muslims alike. Hijama cupping therapy has gone through periods of decline and resurgence, depending on political, social, and scientific circumstances. Some modern medical authorities and practitioners dismissed Hijama cupping treatment as antiquated, unscientific, and hazardous. However, many modern medical researchers and practitioners rediscovered and welcomed Hijama cupping therapy, recognizing its efficacy, safety, and compatibility with other treatments. Hijama cupping treatment has also acquired popularity and acceptability among the broader population, particularly among Muslims and non-Muslims who value natural, holistic, and alternative health. Hijama cupping therapy is currently widely used and promoted in several nations and areas, including the Middle East, Asia, Africa, Europe, America, and Australia.

The modern revival and popularity of hijama cupping therapy

The European Renaissance of Hijama Cupping Therapy

Hijama cupping therapy was adopted and expanded throughout Europe, as proven by the activity of European scholars and physicians who translated and modified Islamic medicinal writings. The Arabs taught Europeans about Hijama cupping therapy, which they acquired and improved from the Prophet Muhammad, who prescribed and conducted cupping for a variety of illnesses. Europeans cupped using glass or metal cups. They would use a syringe or a suction pump to produce a vacuum. They could also utilize scarification, cautery, or medicine to improve the results of cupping.

Some of the famous European scholars and physicians who used Hijama cupping therapy were:

- Paracelsus (1493-1541), the father of toxicology, who used cupping to treat chronic diseases and to remove harmful substances from the body.

- William Harvey (1578-1657), the discoverer of blood circulation, who used cupping to regulate the blood flow and to treat cardiovascular disorders.

- Ambroise Paré (1510-1590), the father of surgery, who used cupping to treat wounds and to prevent infections.

- Franz Anton Mesmer (1734-1815), the founder of

mesmerism, who used cupping to manipulate the magnetic fluid in the body and to cure nervous disorders.

The American Experimentation and Advocacy of Hijama Cupping Therapy

Hijama cupping treatment was used and popularized in America, as proven by the writings of American researchers and physicians who experimented with and promoted the use of cupping. Americans learnt about Hijama cupping therapy from Europeans who introduced the cupping tools and procedures to the New World. Cupping devices used by Americans included glass, metal, and rubber cups. They would utilize a mechanical gadget or a rubber bulb to generate suction. They would also employ antiseptics, antibiotics, or steroids to speed up the cupping healing process.

Some well-known American researchers and physicians who employed Hijama cupping treatment were:

- Benjamin Rush (1746-1813), the father of American medicine, who used cupping to treat yellow fever and to reduce inflammation.

- Edgar Cayce (1877-1945), the sleeping prophet, who used cupping to diagnose and treat various illnesses and to access the subconscious mind.

- Charles Kennedy (1808-1865), the inventor of the cupping scarificator, who used cupping to perform bloodletting and to stimulate the nervous system.

- Arthur Conan Doyle (1859-1930), the creator of Sherlock Holmes, who used cupping to treat his tuberculosis and to relieve his pain.

The Global Resurgence and Promotion of Hijama Cupping Therapy

Hijama cupping treatment was revitalized and spread around the world, as proven by the efforts of modern researchers and physicians who explored and promoted the practice. Modern practitioners of hijama cupping treatment learnt about the advantages and techniques of cupping from a variety of sources, including Islamic teachings, traditional Chinese medicine, scientific research, and personal experience. Modern practitioners employed plastic, silicone, or magnetic cups for cupping. They would produce suction using a vacuum pump or by hand. They would also utilize disposable blades, sterilized equipment, or infrared radiation to improve the safety and effectiveness of cupping.

Some well-known modern scholars and physicians who practiced hijama cupping treatment were:

- The author of The Encyclopedia of Prophetic Medicine, Muhammad Al-Bukhari (1949-present), uses cupping to explain and implement prophetic medicine, as well as to cure numerous maladies.

- Mehmet Oz (1960-present), presenter of The Dr. Oz Show, uses cupping to show and encourage alternative therapy while also improving wellbeing and attractiveness.

- Jennifer Aniston (1969–present), an actress and producer, utilized cupping to ease stress and improve her beauty.

- Michael Phelps (1985–present), a swimmer and Olympian, uses cupping to improve his performance and recuperate from injuries.

History of Hijama

The development of Hijama in the Ottoman Empire

Hijama in the Ottoman Empire was the practice of Hijama

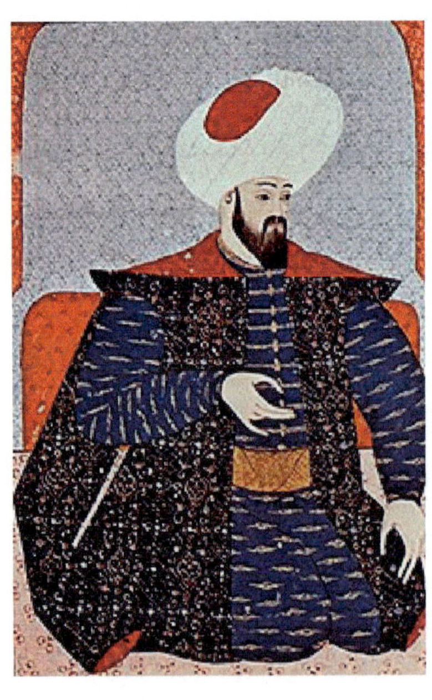

under the reign and influence of the Ottoman Turks, who were Muslims and ancestors of the Mongols and Seljuks. In the Ottoman Empire, Hijama was a component of Islamic medicine, which was founded on the Quran, the Sunnah, and the writings of Muslim intellectuals and physicians such as Ibn Sina, Al-Razi, and Al-Zahrawi. In the Ottoman Empire, Hijama was a common therapy for a variety of ailments and problems, including blood disorders, infections, wounds, and fractures. In the Ottoman Empire, Hijama was a sign of Ottoman culture and identity, as well as a source of pride and dignity for the Ottoman people.

1. The Hijama cannon was invented as a device that used air pressure to generate a vacuum in cups without the need of fire or hand pumping. Hezarfen Ahmet Celebi, a well-known Ottoman pilot and engineer, designed the Hijama gun in the seventeenth century.

2. The Hijama blades were improved by being constructed of high-quality steel and honed to a fine edge, ensuring a clean and accurate cut on the skin. The Hijama blades were also sanitized and cleaned to avoid infection and problems. Serafeddin Sabuncuoglu, a prominent Ottoman surgeon and author, perfected the Hijama blades in the fifteenth century.

3. The introduction of the Hijama chart, a graphic depicting the locations and spots of Hijama on the human body according on organs, ailments, and seasons. The Hijama chart was also provided by thorough instructions and explanations to help both practitioners and patients. Ali bin Isa, a well-known Ottoman ophthalmologist and writer, first devised the Hijama chart in the 14th century.

Hijama in Spain

Hijama was introduced to Spain by Muslims who dominated the Iberian Peninsula from the eighth to the fifteenth centuries. It was widely utilized as a preventative and curative treatment for a variety of ailments, including blood 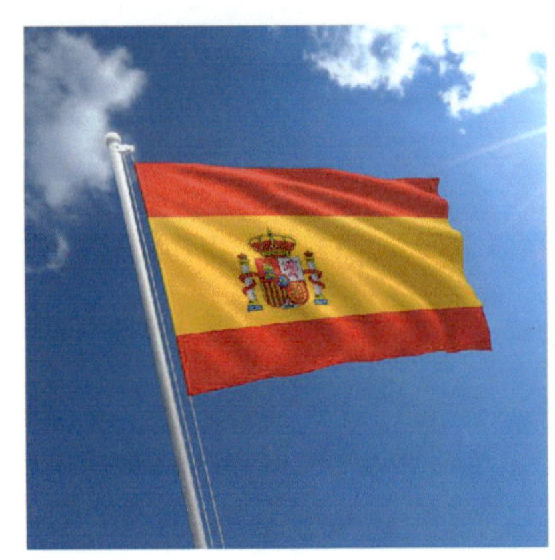 problems. Hijama was also incorporated into other medicinal systems, including Galenic and Unani medicine, which were influenced by Greek and Persian traditions. Hijama's popularity fell following the Reconquista, when Christian nations ousted Muslims from Spain. Some places, like as Andalusia and Catalonia, retained some vestiges of Hijama in their folk medicines.

Hijama in France

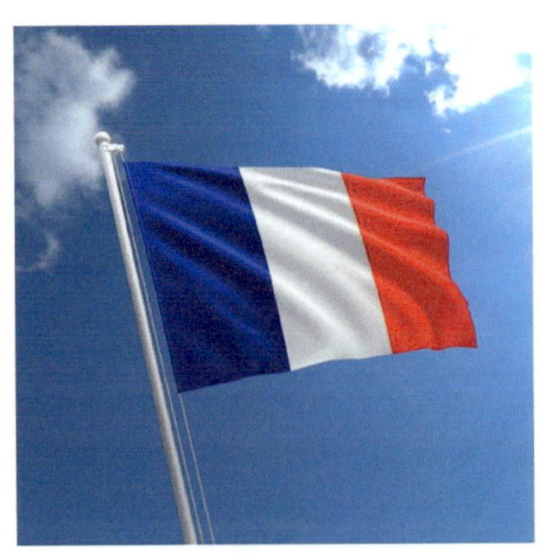 Hijama was known in France as ventouse or sangsue, which translates as cup or leech. It has been used by some physicians and surgeons since the Middle Ages, particularly to treat headaches, migraines, rheumatism, and skin

conditions. Hijama was also employed as a bloodletting procedure, with leeches and lancets, to balance the body's humors. Hijama's popularity declined in the 18th and 19th centuries as new medical theories and practices arose. However, Hijama saw a renaissance in the 20th and 21st centuries, as certain alternative practitioners and communities accepted it as a natural and holistic therapy.

History of Hijama in Germany

In Germany, Hijama was called as Schröpfen or Schröpfkopf, which translates as cupping or cupping head. It has been used by certain physicians and barbers since the medieval period, mostly to relieve pain, inflammation, and congestion. Hijama was 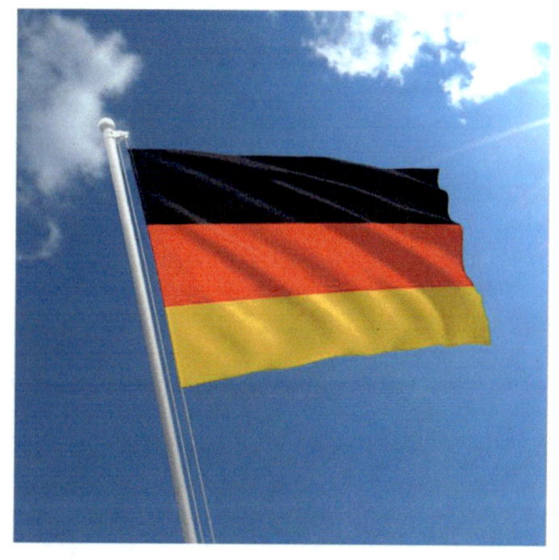 also used for bloodletting, coupled with scarification and leeches, to remove excess blood and fluids from the body. Hijama was influenced by medicinal traditions from Greece, Rome, Persia, and Arabia, and it was combined with other therapies including herbal medicine and hydrotherapy.

Why is Hijama permitted in England, a country that rejects all Islamic values?

Hijama has been utilized for centuries in a variety of civilizations, including England, where it was introduced by

Muslims who governed the Iberian Peninsula from the eighth to the fifteenth centuries.

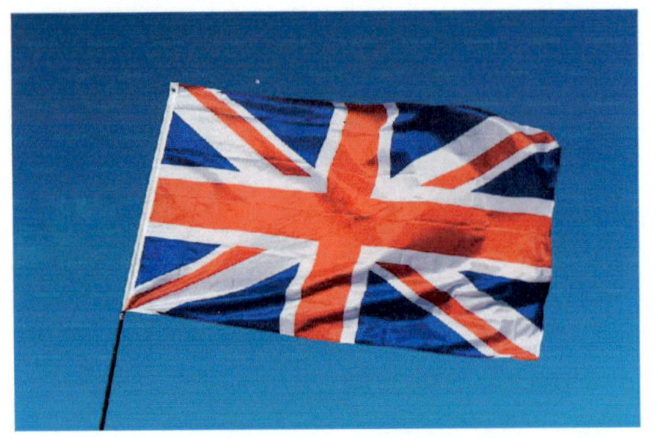

Hijama is allowed in England and other areas of the UK as long as it is performed by certified and registered practitioners who adhere to professional health and safety rules and codes of ethics. Hijama is not governed by a particular law or authority, but it is subject to the basic rules and regulations that apply to other forms of complementary and alternative medicine, including the Human Medicines Regulations 2012, the Health and Safety at Work Act 1974, and the Consumer Protection Act 1987.

Hijama is not against British principles, as the country respects and defends its citizens' and inhabitants' freedom of religion and belief. Hijama is performed by people of many religions and backgrounds, not just Muslims, because it is seen as a natural and comprehensive therapy that may enhance persons' physical and mental health. Hijama is also supported by scientific study and data demonstrating its efficacy and safety for a variety of diseases, including pain, inflammation, infections, and stress.

Hijama in the United States

Hijama has a long and diversified history in the United States, where it was introduced by many immigrants and settlers, including Native Americans, Europeans, Africans, and Asians, who affected the American medical heritage. Hijama 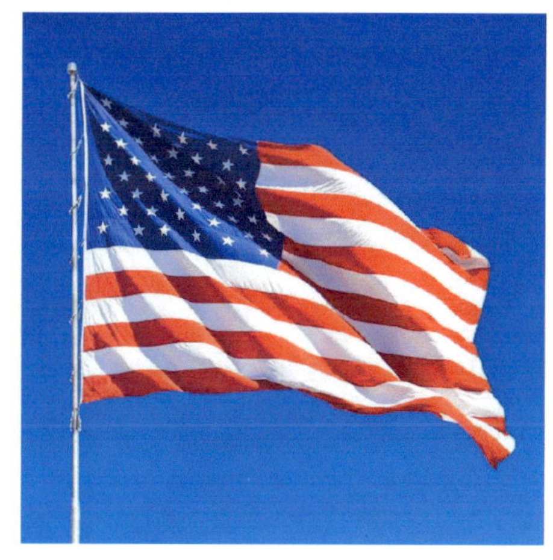 was commonly utilized by American doctors and healers to cure a variety of ailments, including colds, influenza, asthma, and arthritis. Hijama was also popular with Americans, who used it for both medicinal and cosmetic purposes. Hijama was regarded as a simple and successful kind of therapy, and it was performed and advocated in popular American publications and literature.

Hijama in the Netherlands

Hijama was known in the Netherlands as koppen or koppenzetten, which means to cups or cupping. It has been used by certain physicians and surgeons since the 16th century, 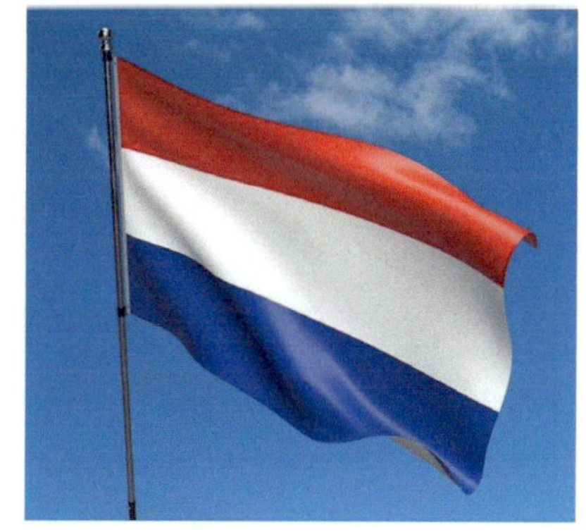

mostly to treat headaches, migraines, neuralgia, and sciatica. Hijama has a long and diverse history in the Netherlands, where it was brought by several cultures and civilizations, including the Romans, Frisians, Saxons, and Arabs, who all affected the Dutch medical tradition. Hijama was widely used by the Dutch physicians and surgeons, who utilized it to cure numerous maladies, such as headaches, gout, infections, and wounds. Hijama was also popular with the Dutch people, who utilized it for its health and beauty benefits.

Hijama was considered as a scientific and sensible technique of therapy, and it was taught and practiced at the Netherlands' prestigious medical schools and hospitals. Hijama has had a renaissance in the Netherlands in the twenty-first century, owing to an increased interest in natural and alternative remedies, as well as the influence of the Muslim community, which considers Hijama as a prophetic and religious activity. Hijama is currently accessible in many cities and areas throughout the Netherlands, where it is provided by trained and competent practitioners who adhere to the rules and regulations of the Dutch Association of Traditional Chinese Medicine.

Hijama in Malaysia

Arab and Indian traders introduced Hijama to Malaysia, bringing with them their medical traditions and practices. It was used by some healers and practitioners from the 15th century, mostly to relieve pain, inflammation, and infection.

Hijama was also utilized as a preventative and curative measure for a variety of ailments, including blood abnormalities. Hijama was influenced by medicinal traditions from Arabia, India, China, and Indonesia, and it was combined

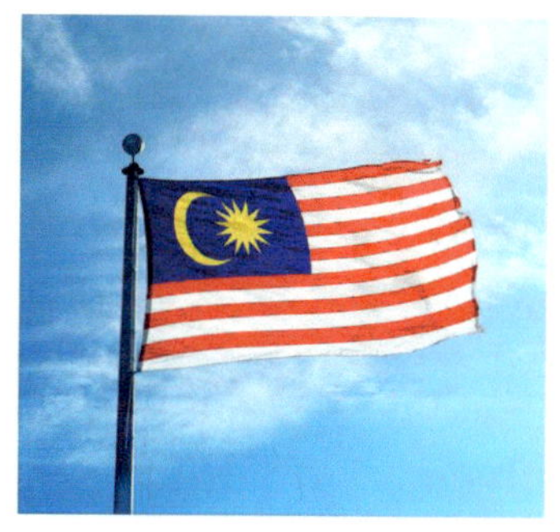

with other therapies including Islamic medicine and Malay medicine. Malay Muslim physicians and intellectuals utilized Hijama to cure a variety of ailments, including fever, asthma, diabetes, and hypertension. Hijama was also popular among Malay Muslims, who utilized it for both health and spiritual reasons.

History of Hijama in Russia

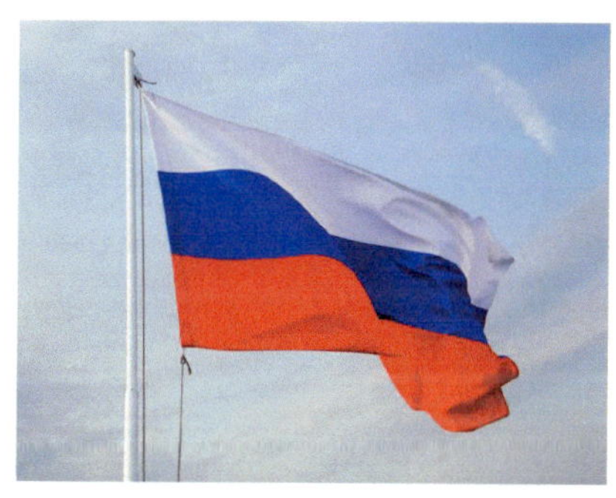

Hijama has a long and varied history in Russia, where it was known by several names, including Schröpfen, Blutegel, and Baunscheidtieren. Hijama was introduced to Russia by different nations and civilizations, including the Romans, Celts, Saxons, Franks, and Arabs, all of whom affected Russian medicinal traditions. Russian doctors and healers used Hijama to treat a variety of disorders, including fever, rheumatism, gout, and neuralgia. Hijama was also popular among the general public, who practiced it at home or in the countryside with basic tools and materials like horns, shells, or glass jars. Hijama has regained some popularity in Russia in the twenty-first century, owing to rising desire for natural and alternative medicines, as well as the existence of the Muslim population, which regards Hijama as a prophetic and spiritual activity. Some qualified and educated practitioners currently practice Hijama in accordance with the regulations and criteria established by the National Certification Commission for Acupuncture and Oriental Medicine. Hijama is also supported by scientific studies and trials that demonstrate its advantages and effects.

History of Hijama in Turkey

Hijama was known in Turkey as hacamat or hacamat tedavisi, which means to cupping or cupping treatment. Hijama has a long and diverse history in Turkey, having been brought by several civilizations and peoples, including the Romans, Mongols, Seljuks, and Ottomans, all of whom affected Turkish medical tradition. Turkish physicians and surgeons commonly employed

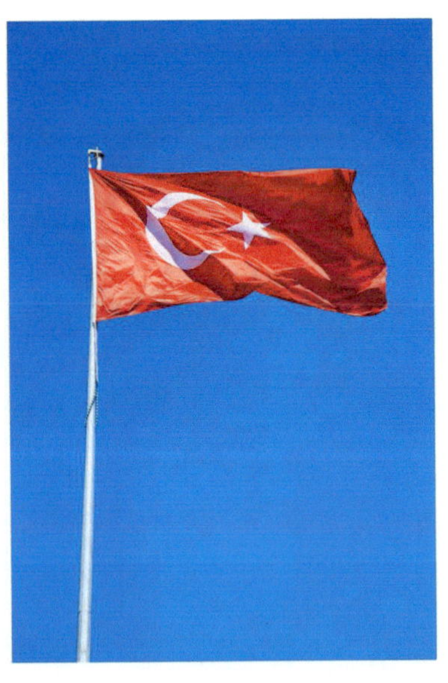

Hijama to cure a variety of ailments, including plague, smallpox, scurvy, and cholera. Hijama was also popular with the Turkish populace, who sought it out for its therapeutic and preventative properties. Hijama was regarded as a scientific and reasonable

therapeutic procedure, and it was taught and performed at Turkey's most famous medical schools and institutes. Hijama is currently accessible in many cities and towns in Turkey, where it is provided by certified and qualified practitioners who adhere to the Turkish Cupping Society's norms and rules. Hijama is also supported by scientific research and evaluations that demonstrate its efficacy and safety.

Hijama Tools Through the Ages: Unraveling the Historical Fabric

Hijama materials are the tools and devices used to perform Hijama, including cups, blades, pumps, and antiseptics. Hijama materials have developed over time to reflect the availability, preferences, and invention of various cultures and places. The history of Hijama materials is separated into three major periods: ancient, medieval, and modern.

The ancient period

Hijama materials were plain and unsophisticated in ancient times. The cups were created out of animal horns, shells, bones, or ceramics. The blades were manufactured from flint, stone, or metal. The pumps were manufactured out of animal skins, leather, or wood. The antiseptics were composed of herbs, oils, or vinegar.

The medieval period

Hijama materials evolved and improved during the medieval period. The cups were fashioned from glass, metal, or bamboo.

The blades were constructed from steel, iron, or brass. The pumps were fashioned from rubber, brass, or glass. The antiseptics were composed of alcohol, honey, or salt.

The modern period

Hijama materials have evolved and modernized over time. The cups were manufactured out of silicone, plastic, or acrylic. The blades were constructed from disposable razors, needles, and lancets. The pumps were made of electric, manual, or magnetic components. The antiseptics contained iodine, hydrogen peroxide, or chlorhexidine.

Chapter 03

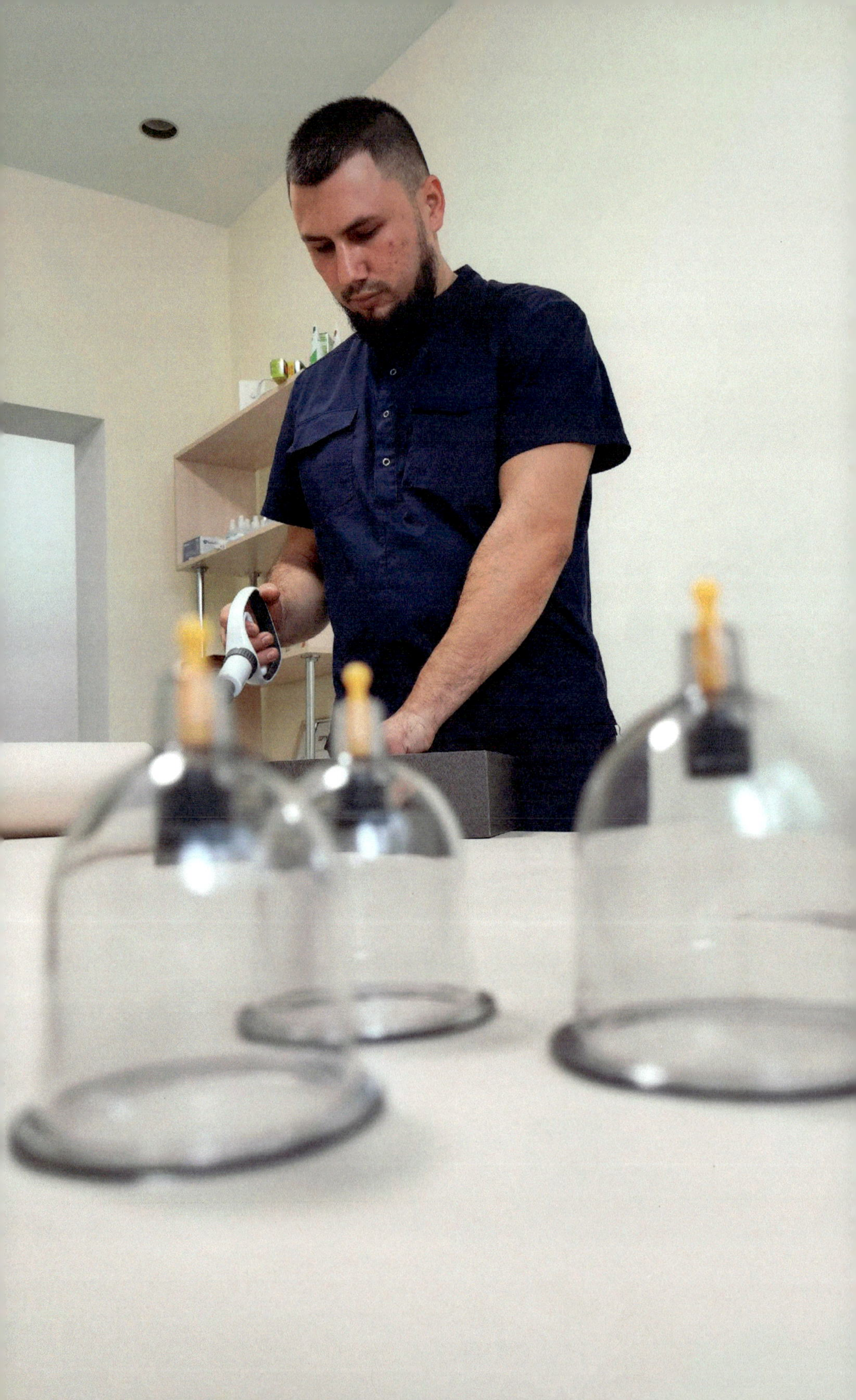

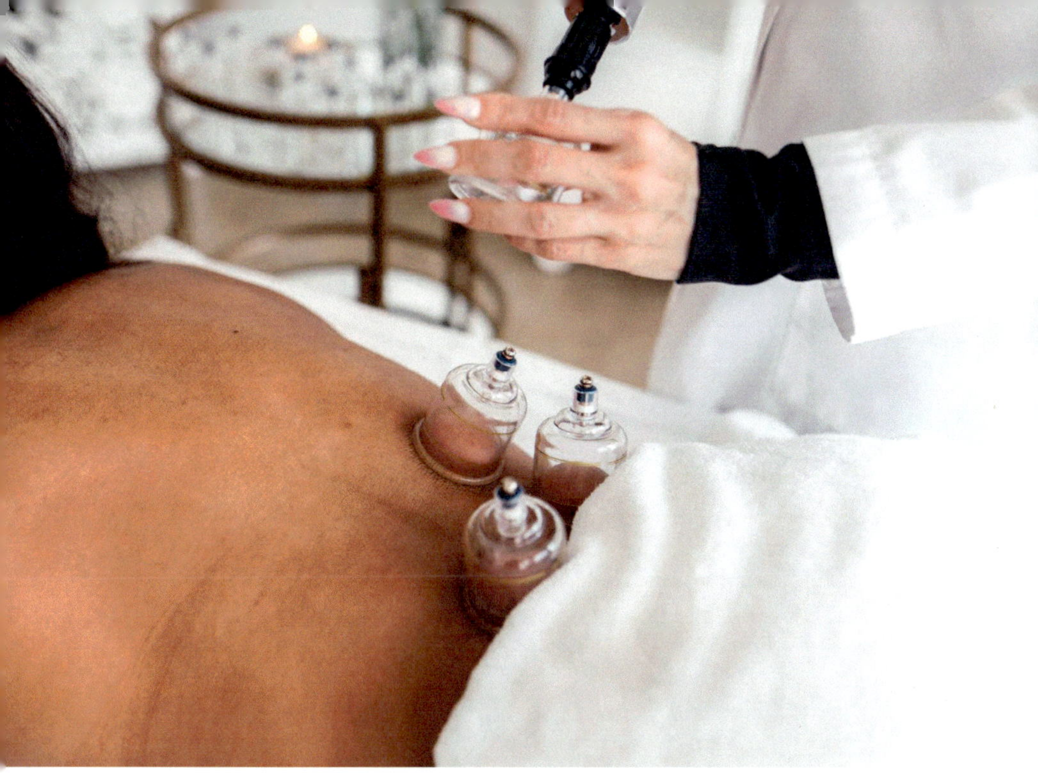

What Are the Different Types and Methods of Hijama Cupping Therapy?

In this chapter, you will study about the different types and techniques of Hijama cupping therapy, such as dry cupping, blood cupping, moving cupping, needle cupping, moxa cupping, empty cupping, full cupping, herbal cupping, and water cupping. You will also learn about the benefits and drawbacks of each type and approach, as well as when and how to apply them effectively. Hijama cupping therapy is an alternative medical technique that includes producing suction on the skin with cups to promote blood flow, eliminate toxins, and balance the body's energy. Hijama cupping therapy is grouped into many types and procedures based on the tools, techniques, and aims of cupping.

Hijama Cupping Therapy Points According to Sunnah

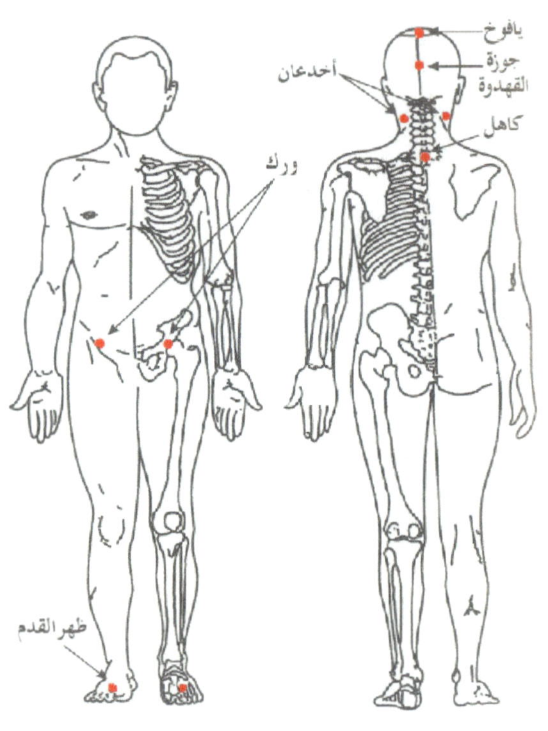

Hijama cupping therapy is a therapeutic technique that includes placing cups on particular locations on the body to create suction and extract blood and fluids. It is based on the Prophet Muhammad's (SAW) teachings and traditions, which endorsed it as a useful and effective cure for a variety of diseases. His distinguished associates (RA) recorded his Hijama-related sayings and actions in the Ahaadeeth volumes, which serve us with important advice and insight on the subject.

One of the things we may learn from the Ahaadeeth is about the Sunnah spots of Hijama, which are the places on the body where the Prophet (SAW) performed Hijama or instructed others to do so. These areas are thought to be the most effective and useful for Hijama because they correspond to the body's major organs, blood arteries, nerves, and energy systems. Hijama has nine Sunnah points, which are listed below:

Yafookh (The Crown Point)

This point is situated at the top of the head, and it is also known as the mother of diseases. It is the first Sunnah point of Hijama, and it is beneficial for treating headaches, migraines, dizziness, insomnia, depression, anxiety, and mental disorders. It also helps to develop memory, concentration, and intelligence. It is reported that the Prophet (SAW) performed Hijama on this point when he was poisoned by a Jewish woman in Khyber.

Abdullah ibn Abbas (R.A) reported that Our Holy Prophet (PBUH) was cupped on his head. Saheeh al Bukhari(5699).

Abdullah ibn Abbas (R.A) also reported that Messenger (PBUH) was cupped on his head for a severe headache while He was in Ihraam. Sahih al-Bukhari (5701).

Al-Akhda'ain (The Posterior Jugulars)

These points are situated at the back of the neck, under the hairline, on the right and left sides. They are the second and third Sunnah points of Hijama, and they

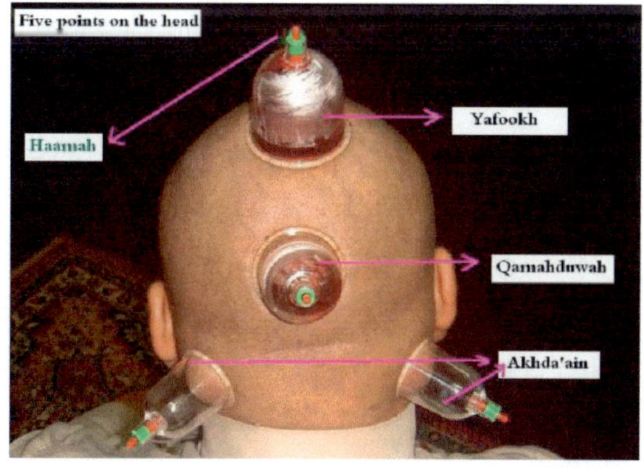

are beneficial for treating ear, nose, and throat problems,

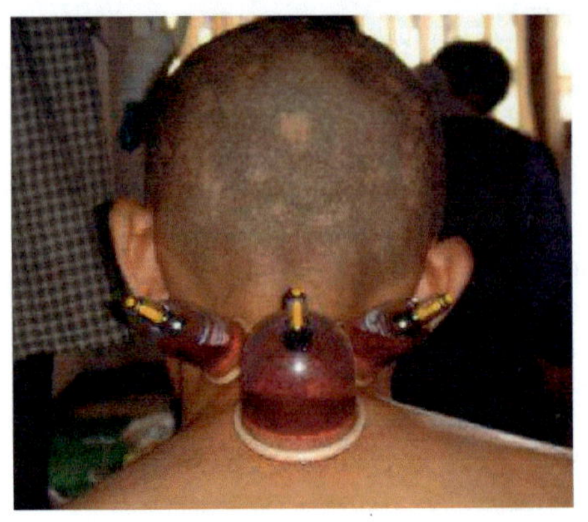

such as earache, tinnitus, sinusitis, sore throat, and tonsillitis. They also aid to relieve neck pain, stiffness, and tension. It is reported that the Prophet (SAW) performed hijama on these points when he was advised by Angel Jibreel.

Anas bin Maalik (may Allah be pleased with him) reported that The Messenger (PBUH) was treated with cupping 3 times on the two veins on the side of the neck and the base of the neck. Saheeh Sunan Abi Dawud (3860), Sunnah ibn Majjal (3483).

Al-Kahil (The Upper Back)

This point is situated between the shoulder blades, and it is the fourth Sunnah point of Hijama. It is useful for treating respiratory problems, such as asthma, bronchitis, cough, and cold. It also helps to improve blood circulation, immune system, and heart function. It is reported that the Prophet (SAW) performed Hijama on this point three times when he was poisoned by a Jewish woman in Khyber.

Narrated by Ibn Majah, the angel Jibreel advised Prophet (PBUH) to perform Hijama on Akhda'ain and al-kahil.

Abdullah bin bauhinia (r.a) reported that our Prophet (PBUH) took Hijama on Haamah and between the shoulders (Al-Kahil).

Al-Katifain (The Shoulders)

These points are situated on the right and left sides of the fourth point, and they are the fifth and sixth Sunnah points of Hijama. They are beneficial for treating muscular and skeletal pains, such as back pain, shoulder pain, arthritis, and rheumatism. They also help to reduce stress, fatigue, and inflammation. It is reported that the Prophet (SAW) performed Hijama on these points when he was suffering from a debilitation.

Al-Waraq (The Waist)

These points are situated on the right and left sides of the lower back, and they are the seventh and eighth Sunnah points of Hijama. They are useful for treating urinary and digestive problems, such as kidney stones, bladder infections, constipation, and diarrhea. They also aid to relieve lower back pain, sciatica, and menstrual cramps. It is reported that the Prophet (SAW) performed Hijama on these points when he was suffering from a pain in his hip.

Jaabir Ibn Abdullah (r.a) reported that Rasool Allah (PBUH) was cupped on his hips for pain relief in that area.

Al-Qadamein (The Feet)

These points are situated on the top of the feet, and they are the ninth Sunnah point of Hijama. They are advantageous for treating swelling, edema, gout, and varicose veins. They also help to stimulate the reflexology zones of the feet, which correspond to different organs and systems of the body. It is reported that the Prophet (SAW) executed Hijama on these points when he was in a state of Ihram during his journey to Makkah.

Jaabir Ibn Abdullah reported that the Messenger (PBUH) fell from his horse onto the trunk of the palm tree and dislocated his foot, so He was cupped on the bruising. Saheeh Sunan Ibn Majah (2807). Anas Ibn Maalik said, "Our dear Prophet (PBUH) was cupped on the top of his foot". Sahheh Sunan Ibn Dawud (1836)

Al-Qamahduwah (The Nape Cavity)

This point is situated at the base of the skull, where the neck meets the head. It is the tenth Sunnah point of Hijama, and it is advantageous for treating nervous system disorders, such as epilepsy, paralysis, stroke, and Parkinson's disease. It also helps to relieve headaches, migraines, insomnia, and stress. It is reported that the Prophet (SAW) said: "Use Hijama (wet cupping) on the qamahduwah (above the nape cavity), for it cures seventy-two kinds of ailments." (Narrated by Tabraani).

Al-Mughayyam (The Knees)

These points are situated on the right and left sides of the knees, and they are the 11th and 12th Sunnah points of Hijama. They are useful for treating joint and bone problems, such as arthritis, rheumatism, osteoporosis, and gout. They also help to improve mobility, flexibility, and strength.

Al-Akhdhayn (The Ankles)

These points are situated on the right and left sides of the ankles, and they are the 13th and 14th Sunnah points of Hijama. They are beneficial for treating foot and leg problems, such as swelling, edema, varicose veins, and cramps. They also aid to stimulate the reflexology zones of the feet, which correspond to different organs and systems of the body.

Types of Hijama cupping therapy

Dry cupping

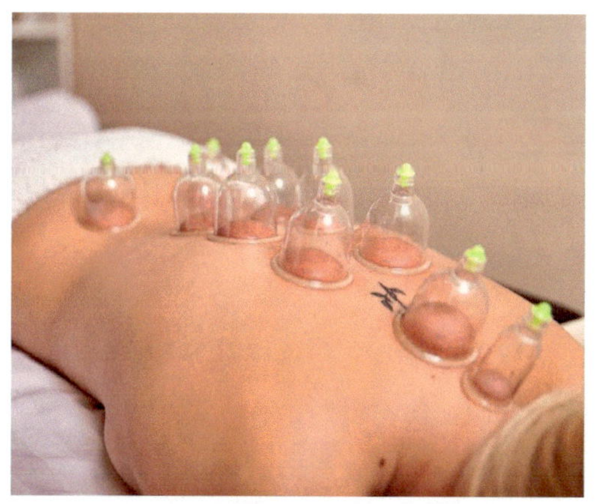

Dry cupping is a type of Hijama cupping therapy that involves placing suction cups on the skin without making any incisions. Dry cupping can provide a number of health and wellness advantages, including increased blood circulation, muscle relaxation, and nerve stimulation. Dry cupping can also be used to prevent and diagnose illnesses, identifying areas of imbalance or blockage in the system.

The procedure for dry cupping is as follows:

- Prepare the patient, cups, and the cupping area. The patient should be in a comfortable, relaxed position, such as lying down or sitting. The cups should be clean, sterile, and the appropriate size and shape. The cupped area should be exposed, clean, and dry.

- Choose a method for creating suction. Suction can be created using a variety of methods, including fire, pumps, and rubber bulbs. The approach should be appropriate for the patient and the situation, and it should be carried out correctly and safely.

- Apply the cups to your skin. Cups should be placed on specific areas of the body, such as the back, neck, shoulders, or legs. The cups should be properly secured to the skin, but not unduly tight or loose. The number and duration of the cups varies depending on the patient and their condition, but they usually range from 3 to 15 cups and 5 to 15 minutes.

- Remove the cups from your skin. The cups should be withdrawn gently and carefully, either by releasing the suction or lowering the cup edges. Clean and disinfect the cups after each use.

- Observe and analyze the results. The color, shape, and texture of the skin, as well as the cup markings, show the results of dry cupping. The findings can be assessed using the patient's symptoms, indicators, and emotions, as well as the condition.

- Some of the benefits of dry cupping include:

- It is straightforward, safe, and painless because it does not involve bleeding or cutting.

- It is safe for most people because there are no notable contraindications or side effects.

- It is versatile, as it can be used on many parts of the body and in conjunction with other treatments.

Wet cupping

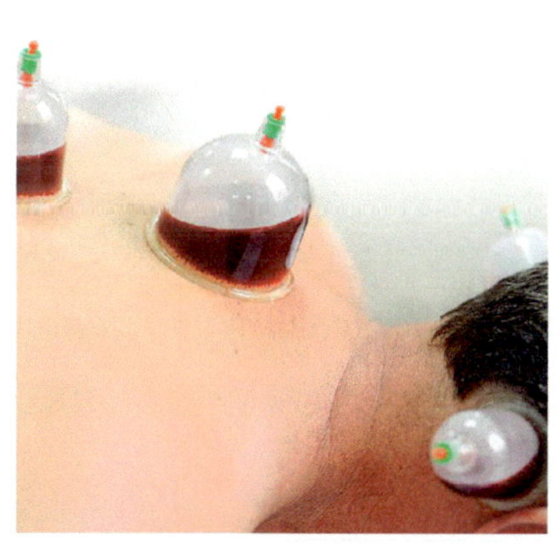

Wet cupping is a sort of Hijama cupping therapy that includes placing suction cups on the skin after making minor incisions. Wet cupping can treat a variety of ailments and disorders, including blood stasis, toxins, and pathogens, as well as discomfort, inflammation, and infection. Wet cupping can also be used for purification and detoxification, since it can rid the blood and body of toxic substances.

The process for wet cupping is as follows:

- Prepare the patient, the cups, the blades, and the area for cupping. The patient should be in a comfortable and relaxed position, such as lying down or sitting. The patient must also be informed and consented to the treatment, and there should be no contraindications or precautions for blood cupping. The cups should be clean, antiseptic, and the proper size and form. The blades should be sharp, disposable, and sterilized. The cupped region should be exposed, clean, and dry.

- Apply the cups to your skin. Cups should be put on certain locations or parts of the body, such as the back, neck, shoulders, or legs. The cups should be securely fastened to the skin, but not overly tight or too loose. The number and duration of the cups vary according to the patient and condition, but they typically range from 3 to 15 cups and 3 to 5 minutes.

- Remove the cups from your skin. The cups should be removed softly and slowly, either by releasing the suction or lowering the cups' edges. The cups should be cleaned and disinfected after each use.

- Make tiny incisions into the skin. Using the blades, make incisions at the same spots or areas where the cups were applied. The incisions should be shallow, tiny, and evenly spaced, with no considerable bleeding or pain. The blades should be disposed of properly after usage.

- Reapply the cups to your skin. The cups should be reapplied to the same locations or areas where the incisions were made, with the same way of establishing suction. The cups should be securely fastened to the skin, but not overly tight or too loose. The number and duration of the cups vary according to the patient and condition, but they typically range from 3 to 15 cups and 10 to 20 minutes.

- Remove the cups from your skin. The cups should be removed softly and slowly, either by releasing the suction or lowering the cups' edges. The cups should be cleaned and disinfected after each use.

- Observe and analyze the outcomes. Blood cupping results can be seen in the amount, color, and quality of blood and fluids removed from the body and collected in cups. The results can be evaluated based on the patient's symptoms, indicators, and sentiments, as well as the condition.

Some of the advantages of wet cupping include:

- It is more effective, medicinal, and purifying because it eliminates stagnant or unclean blood and fluids from the body.

- It is targeted, tailored, and individualized, as it can be applied to specific places or sections of the body according on the patient's diagnosis and needs.

- It is holistic, comprehensive, and integrative because it may address the disease's underlying causes and symptoms while also improving the patient's physical, mental, and spiritual health.

Glide cupping

Glide cupping is a type of Hijama cupping therapy in which suction cups are applied to the skin and moved along 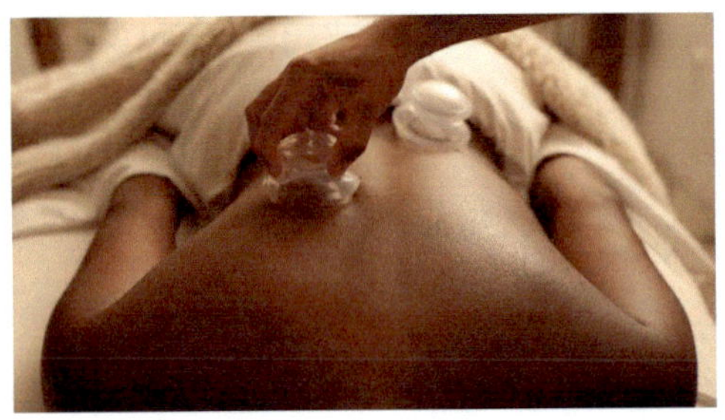 meridians or parts of the body. Glide cupping can be used to massage and relax by loosening the fascia, enhancing range of motion, and lowering stress. Glide cupping can also be used to stimulate and activate the body by improving blood and lymph circulation, as well as invigorating energy and metabolism.

The process for glide cupping is as follows:

- Prepare the patient, the cups, the lubricant, and the area for cupping. The patient should be in a comfortable and relaxed position, such as lying down or sitting. The cups should be clean, antiseptic, and the proper size and form. The lubricant should be natural, organic, and safe for the skin and body, such as an oil, cream, or gel. The cupped region should be exposed, clean, and dry.

- Apply lubricant to your skin. The lubricant should be administered to certain places or areas on the body, such as the back, neck, shoulders, or legs. The lubricant should be sufficient to reduce friction and resistance while not interfering with suction and stimulation levels.

- Apply the cups to your skin. The cups should be put on particular points or sections of the body, using the same suction-creating technique as dry cupping. The cups should be securely fastened to the skin, but not overly tight or too loose. The amount and duration of the cups vary depending on the patient and the condition, but they typically range from one to three cups and ten to thirty minutes.

- Slide the cups across the skin. The cups should be moved down the body's meridians, which include the spine, shoulders, arms, and legs. The direction, speed, and pressure of the sliding vary according on the patient and the disease, but they typically follow the natural flow of blood and energy and are mild and consistent. The sliding should be done gently and smoothly, with little pain or discomfort.

- Remove the cups from your skin. The cups should be removed softly and slowly, either by releasing the suction or lowering the cups' edges. The cups should be cleaned and disinfected after each use.

- Observe and analyze the outcomes. The color, shape, and texture of the skin, as well as the cup markings, reveal the consequences of movement cupping. The results can be evaluated based on the patient's symptoms, indicators, and sentiments, as well as the condition.

Some of the advantages of glide cupping include:

- It is more dynamic, flexible, and calming since it applies a constant and moderate pressure and movement to the skin and muscles.

- It is more efficient, convenient, and cost-effective because it requires fewer cups and takes less time and space to complete.

- It is more comfortable, pleasant, and fulfilling since it provides a warm and relaxing experience as well as smooth and soft skin.

Moxa cupping

Moxa cupping is a type of Hijama cupping therapy that includes placing suction cups on the skin after burning Moxa (dried mugwort) within them. Moxa cupping can be used to warm and tonify the body, such as removing cold and dampness, strengthening the yang, and increasing immunity. Moxa cupping can also be used to treat cold and deficiency-related illnesses like arthritis, asthma, and diarrhea.

The process for Moxa cupping is as follows:

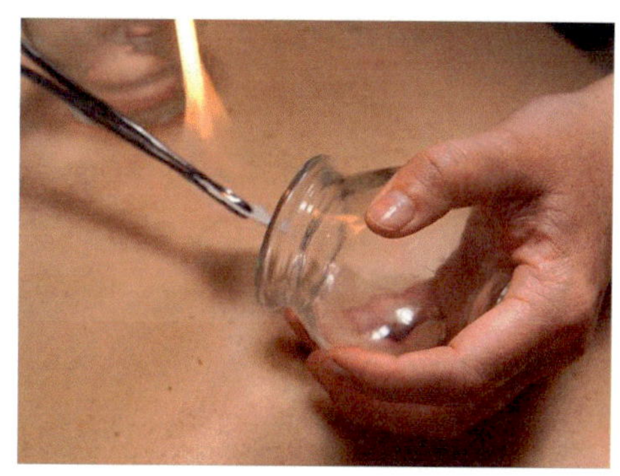

- Prepare the patient, the cups, the Moxa, and the cupping arca. The patient should be in a comfortable and relaxed position, such as lying down or sitting. The patient must also be informed and consented to the process, and there should be no contraindications or precautions for Moxa cupping. The cups should be clean, antiseptic, and the proper size and form. The Moxa should be natural, organic, and of high quality, such as sticks, cones, or wool. The cupped region should be exposed, clean, and dry.

- Light the Moxa and place it in the cups. Light the Moxa with a lighter or match and place it inside the cups, either directly or indirectly. Direct Moxa cupping involves applying the Moxa directly to the skin and then covering it with a cup. Indirect Moxa cupping entails laying the Moxa on a medium, such as ginger, garlic, or salt, then applying the medium to the skin and covering it with a cup. The number and duration of the Moxa vary according to the patient and the situation, but it typically ranges from 1 to 3 pieces and 5 to 15 minutes.

- Apply the cups to your skin. The cups should be put on specific locations or parts of the body, such as the back, abdomen, chest, or legs. The cups should be securely fastened to the skin, but not overly tight or too loose. The number and duration of the cups vary according to the patient and condition, but they typically range from 3 to 15 cups and 10 to 30 minutes.

- Remove the cups from your skin. The cups should be removed softly and slowly, either by releasing the suction or lowering the cups' edges. The cups should be cleaned and disinfected after each use. Following use, the Moxa and medium should be carefully disposed of.

- Observe and analyze the outcomes. The warmth, color, and texture of the skin and tissues are indicators of Moxa cupping's effectiveness. The results can be evaluated based on the patient's symptoms, indicators, and sentiments, as well as the condition.

Some of the benefits of Moxa cupping include:

- It is more warm, nourishing, and revitalizing because it incorporates the thermal and herbal characteristics of Moxa into the suction and stimulation of cupping.

- It is more suited for persons with a cold or weak constitution because it warms and energizes the body and organs.

- It is more helpful for chronic or resistant ailments since it can go deeper and continue longer than other forms of cupping.

Full cupping

Full cupping is a type of Hijama cupping therapy that involves placing suction cups on the skin after filling them with water, oil, honey, or herbs. Full cupping can be used to enhance the

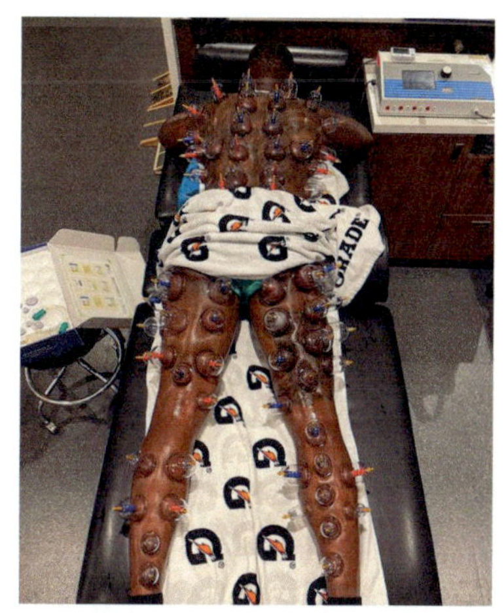

skin's qualities and functions, such as cleansing, hydrating, nurturing, and healing. Full cupping can also be used to treat skin diseases like acne, eczema, and wounds that require topical or local treatment.

The process for full cupping is as follows:

• Prepare the patient, the cups, the substances, and the area for cupping. The patient should be in a comfortable and relaxed position, such as lying down or sitting. The patient must also be informed and consented to the procedure, and there should be no contraindications or precautions for thorough cupping. The cups should be clean, antiseptic, and the proper size and form. Water, oil, honey, vinegar, or herbs are all examples of natural, organic, and skin and body-friendly ingredients. The cupped region should be exposed, clean, and dry.

- Fill each cup with the substances. The substances should be poured into the cups, either partially or completely, depending on the intended effect and quantity. The substances should be at the appropriate temperature, consistency, and quality, and they should not cause harm or pain to the patient or the skin.

- Apply the cups to your skin. Cups should be placed on specific locations or parts of the body, such as the face, chest, back, or legs. The cups should be securely fastened to the skin, but not overly tight or too loose. The number and duration of the cups vary according to the patient and condition, but they typically range from 3 to 15 cups and 10 to 30 minutes.

- Remove the cups from your skin. The cups should be removed softly and slowly, either by releasing the suction or lowering the cups' edges. The cups should be cleaned and disinfected after each use. The substances should be removed or washed from the skin.

- Observe and analyze the outcomes. The appearance, condition, and sensation of the skin and tissues can be used to assess the effectiveness of full cupping. The results can be evaluated based on the patient's symptoms, indicators, and sentiments, as well as the condition.

Some of the benefits of complete cupping include:

- It is more diverse, tailored, and holistic since it can use a variety of substances and combinations to meet the needs and preferences of the patient and condition.

- It is more useful to the skin since it can hydrate, nourish, protect, and regenerate the skin and tissues.

- It is more beneficial for external or superficial ailments because it has direct effects on the skin and body's surface.

Herbal cupping

Herbal cupping is a type of Hijama cupping therapy that involves placing suction cups on the skin after soaking them

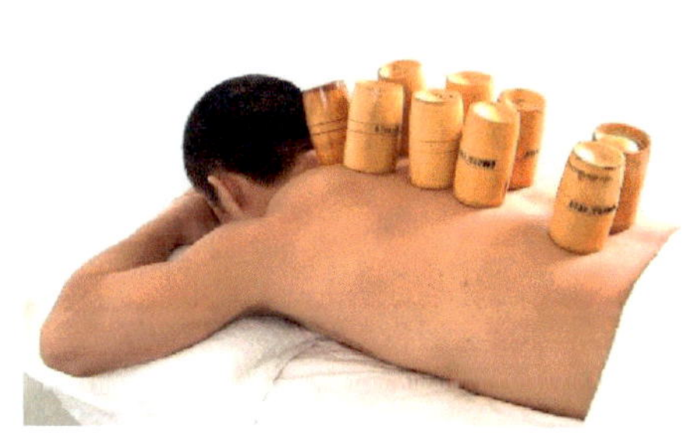

in herbal decoctions or infusions. Herbal cupping can be used to incorporate herbal medicine benefits such as organ, system, and elemental harmony, as well as treating various imbalances and diseases. Herbal cupping can also be utilized to enhance the effects of cupping by combining the medicinal and therapeutic characteristics of herbs with cupping's suction and stimulation.

The process for herbal cupping is as follows:

- Prepare the patient, the cups, the herbs, and the area for cupping. The patient should be in a comfortable and relaxed position, such as lying down or sitting. The patient must also be informed and consented to the process, and there should be no contraindications or precautions for herbal cupping. The cups should be clean, antiseptic, and the proper size and form. Herbs should be natural, organic, and of high quality, and they should be selected, processed, and used in accordance with herbal medicine principles and theories. The cupped region should be exposed, clean, and dry.

- Soak the cups in your herbal decoctions or infusions. Herbal decoctions or infusions should be prepared by boiling or steeping the herbs in water at the appropriate temperature, concentration, and amount. Soak the cups in the herbal decoctions or infusions for a few minutes, until completely saturated and heated.

- Apply the cups to your skin. Cups should be placed on specific locations or parts of the body, such as the back, chest, abdomen, or limbs. The cups should be securely fastened to the skin, but not overly tight or too loose. The number and duration of the cups vary according to the patient and condition, but they typically range from 3 to 15 cups and 10 to 30 minutes.

- Remove the cups from your skin. The cups should

be removed softly and slowly, either by releasing the suction or lowering the cups' edges. The cups should be cleaned and disinfected after each use.

- Observe and analyze the outcomes. The scent, color, and texture of the skin and tissues indicate the results of herbal cupping. The results can be evaluated based on the patient's symptoms, indicators, and sentiments, as well as the condition.

Some of the benefits of herbal cupping include:

- It is more natural, organic, and compatible because it contains plant-derived herbs that are beneficial to both the body and nature.

- It is more thorough and integrative since it can treat the entire body, including the physical, mental, emotional, and spiritual elements of the patient and the ailment.

- It is more particular and successful since it can employ different herbs and formulas based on the patient's diagnosis and treatment of the ailment.

Water cupping

Water cupping is a type of Hijama cupping therapy that includes placing suction cups on the skin after filling them with water. Water cupping can be used to create hydrostatic pressure and a vacuum effect, which can help draw out more blood and toxins while also boosting suction and stimulation. Water cupping can also be used to treat heat-related disorders,

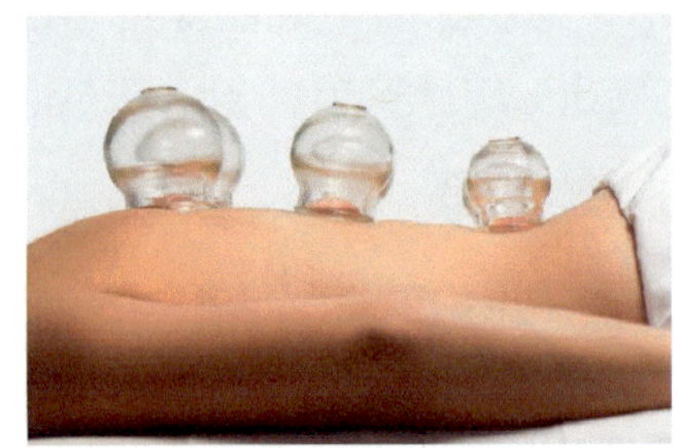

such as fever, hypertension, or edema, which require cooling or draining.

The process for water cupping is as follows:

- Prepare the patient, the cups, the water, and the cupping area. The patient should be in a comfortable and relaxed position, such as lying down or sitting. The patient must also be informed and consented to the process, and there should be no contraindications or precautions for water cupping. The cups should be clean, antiseptic, and the proper size and form. The water should be clean, pure, and at the appropriate temperature, whether cold, warm, or hot, depending on the desired effect and the patient's tolerance level. The cupped region should be exposed, clean, and dry.

- Fill each cup with water. Water should be filled into the cups, either partially or completely, depending on the desired effect and quantity. Pour the water gently and carefully, avoiding spills and splashes.

- Apply the cups to your skin. Cups should be placed on specific locations or parts of the body, such as the back, chest, abdomen, or limbs. The cups should be securely fastened to the skin, but not overly tight or too loose.

The number and duration of the cups vary according to the patient and condition, but they typically range from 3 to 15 cups and 10 to 30 minutes.

- Remove the cups from your skin. The cups should be removed softly and slowly, either by releasing the suction or lowering the cups' edges. The cups should be cleaned and disinfected after each use. Water should be safely drained or collected after usage.

- Observe and analyze the outcomes. Water cupping results can be seen in the amount, color, and quality of blood and fluids removed from the body and collected in cups. The results can be evaluated based on the patient's symptoms, indicators, and sentiments, as well as the condition.

Some of the benefits of water cupping include:

- It is more intense, deep, and purifying because it generates stronger and longer-lasting suction and stimulation while also removing more blood and fluids from the body.

- It is more suited to persons with a heated or excessive constitution since it cools and calms the body and organs.

- It is more effective for acute or severe conditions since it can bring immediate and significant relief and improvement.

Leech Cupping: An Alternative Form of Hijama

Leech cupping is a type of Hijama that utilizes leeches rather than cups to create suction and draw blood from the skin. Leeches are little, worm-like animals that feed on blood 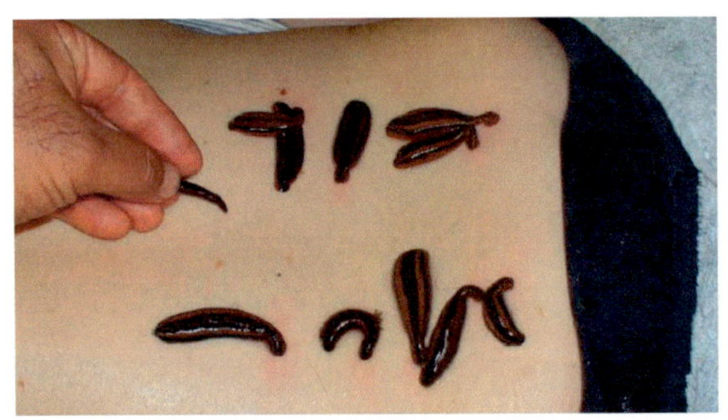 and produce saliva containing a variety of compounds that impact the blood and body. Leech cupping is often referred to as hirudo therapy, derived from the Latin word hirudo, which means leech.

Leech cupping has a long history of use in various civilizations and places, including ancient Egypt, India, Arabia, Greece, Europe, and Asia. It was used to cure a variety of ailments, including skin diseases, dental issues, nervous system disorders, inflammation, and more. Some medical experts and alternative practitioners continue to perform leech cupping, claiming that it has numerous benefits and advantages over conventional cupping.

How Leech Cupping Works

Leech cupping is the process of putting live leeches to particular places on the body, where they adhere and suck blood from capillaries and interstitial fluids. The leeches can be applied to inflamed or afflicted areas, such as the trachea for bronchitis or the ear for earache. The leeches can also be used on the Sunnah points, which are identical to the cupping sites indicated by the Prophet (SAW).

The leeches linger on the skin for 10 to 30 minutes, depending on their size and number, as well as how much blood they drink. During this period, the leeches release their saliva into the wound, which contains a complex mixture of substances, including:

- Local anesthetic: This reduces pain and allows the leech to feed without being noticed. It has a similar structure to natural morphine.

- Local vasodilator: This increases blood flow and enhances the suction of the leech. It also helps to remove toxins and impurities from the blood and the tissues.

- Anticoagulant agents (hirudin): These prevent blood clotting and prolong bleeding. They also prevent thrombosis and improve blood circulation.

- Platelet aggregation inhibitors (calin): These prevent platelets from sticking together and forming clots. They also reduce inflammation and swelling.

Leech saliva also contains a wide range of other substances, including proteins, peptides, hormones, and enzymes, all of which have different effects on the body and blood. Scientists are still finding and researching some of these compounds. The leeches remove themselves from the skin and are disposed of properly once they have finished feeding. The prolonged bleeding of the wound aids in the body's removal of poisons and pollutants. After that, the wound is cleaned, bandaged, and treated with an antiseptic. Usually, the wound heals in a few days, leaving a faint mark.

Benefits of Leech Cupping

Leech cupping is said to have many benefits for the body and the mind, such as:

- Improving blood circulation and oxygenation

- Stimulating the immune system and the lymphatic system

- Relieving pain and inflammation

- Treating various diseases and disorders, such as arthritis, diabetes, hypertension, migraine, eczema, psoriasis, acne, herpes, and more

- Enhancing mood and well-being

- Breaking the effects of evil eye, magic, and jinn possession

Leech cupping also has some advantages over conventional cupping, such as:

- Being more precise and targeted

- Being more gentle and less painful

- Being more effective and efficient

- Being more natural and organic

Leech cupping should only be performed by professional and competent practitioners who utilize sterile and disposable leeches and practice good cleanliness and safeguards. Leech cupping should not be performed on persons with bleeding disorders, low blood pressure, anemia, a weakened immune system, pregnancy, menstruation, or a leech allergy. Leech cupping should not be used on locations with significant blood arteries, nerves, bones, or organs.

How to Prepare Yourself for Hijama

Hijama therapy is a useful and effective way to improve both physical and mental health. To prepare for Hijama, you need

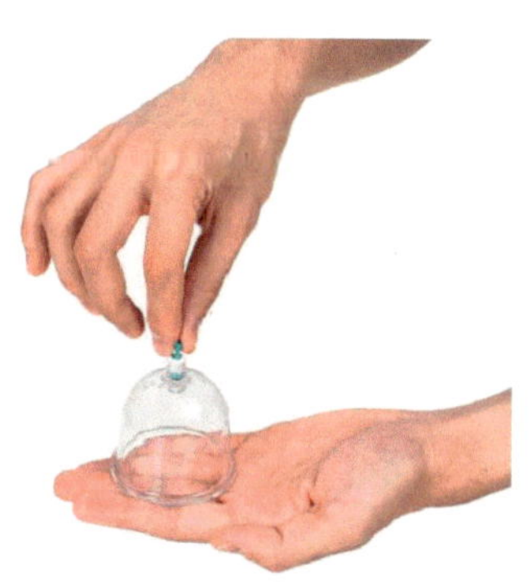

follow some rules and tips before beginning therapy. Here are some of the crucial aspects to consider before Hijama:

Avoid consuming too much or too little.

Eating too much or too little before Hijama is not suggested because it can disrupt blood flow and digestion. Eating too much can leave the stomach full and bloated, interfering with the Hijama process and causing discomfort. Eating too little might leave the body weak and hungry, reducing the effectiveness of the Hijama therapy and causing disorientation. It is recommended that you eat a light and healthy meal and drink plenty of water before Hijama, but cease at least 3 to 4 hours before the treatment.

Avoid eating animal products.

It is recommended that you avoid eating animal products such meat, dairy, or eggs at least 24 hours before Hijama since they can impact the quality and amount of your blood. Animal products may contain hormones, antibiotics, or poisons that might pollute and thicken the blood. This can limit blood circulation and oxygen availability, resulting in increased inflammation and infection. Plant-based meals, such as fruits, vegetables, grains, or nuts, should be consumed before Hijama since they can cleanse and thin the blood.

Avoid any sexual activity.

Sexual activity, such as intercourse or masturbation, should be avoided 24 hours before Hijama since it can alter the body's energy and equilibrium. Sexual activity can drain critical fluids and nutrients, compromising the immune system and the healing process. Sexual activity can also boost hormones and emotions, disrupting the body's sense of peace and relaxation. It is recommended that sexual activity be avoided prior to Hijama in order to maintain the body's vitality and equilibrium.

How to Choose the Best Materials for Hijama (Vacuum Materials)?

Hijama requires the necessary materials to function securely and successfully. The materials for Hijama include cups, devices, instruments, and substances. Materials should be chosen according to their quality, compatibility, and availability. Some elements that can influence the choosing of materials for Hijama include:

- The practitioner or patient's preferred type and method of Hijama.

- The size and shape of the Hijama points that are treated or chosen by the practitioner or patient

- The practitioner or the patient apply or regulate the temperature and pressure of the Hijama technique.

- The cost and convenience of the items that are available or accessible to the practitioner or the patient

How to Enhance the Benefits of Hijama with Simple Tips?

Hijama therapy is a good and effective method of improving both physical and mental health. However, you may maximize the benefits of Hijama by following a few simple recommendations to prepare and care for yourself before, during, and after the treatment. Here are some of the tips that can enhance the benefits of Hijama:

Keep yourself hydrated and nourished.

Hydration and nourishment are essential before and after Hijama since they can help you replenish your energy and hydration levels. Hijama might cause some blood loss, leaving you dehydrated and weak. You should drink plenty of water and consume dates or honey before and after performing Hijama to replenish your natural sugar and mineral reserves. You should also avoid dairy, red meat, and processed foods for at least 24 hours before and after wearing Hijama, as they can strain your digestive and detoxifying systems.

Relax and take long breaths.

Relaxation and deep breathing are essential during and after Hijama since they can help relieve stress and pain. Hijama can produce discomfort and anxiety, affecting blood pressure and heart rate. Relax and breathe deeply during and after Hijama to calm your nerves and muscles. You should also avoid any distractions or disturbances during and after Hijama because they can interfere with your concentration and relaxation.

Cleanse and treat your wounds

Cleaning and dressing your wounds after Hijama is critical to preventing infection and complications. Hijama can cause small, shallow cuts in your skin, exposing it to germs and bacteria. Hijama can protect your skin and incisions from infection and irritation, so clean and dress them afterward. To clean your wounds, use a disinfectant like alcohol, iodine, or hydrogen peroxide, and then apply an ointment like olive oil, black sesame oil, or honey to treat them.

Chapter 04

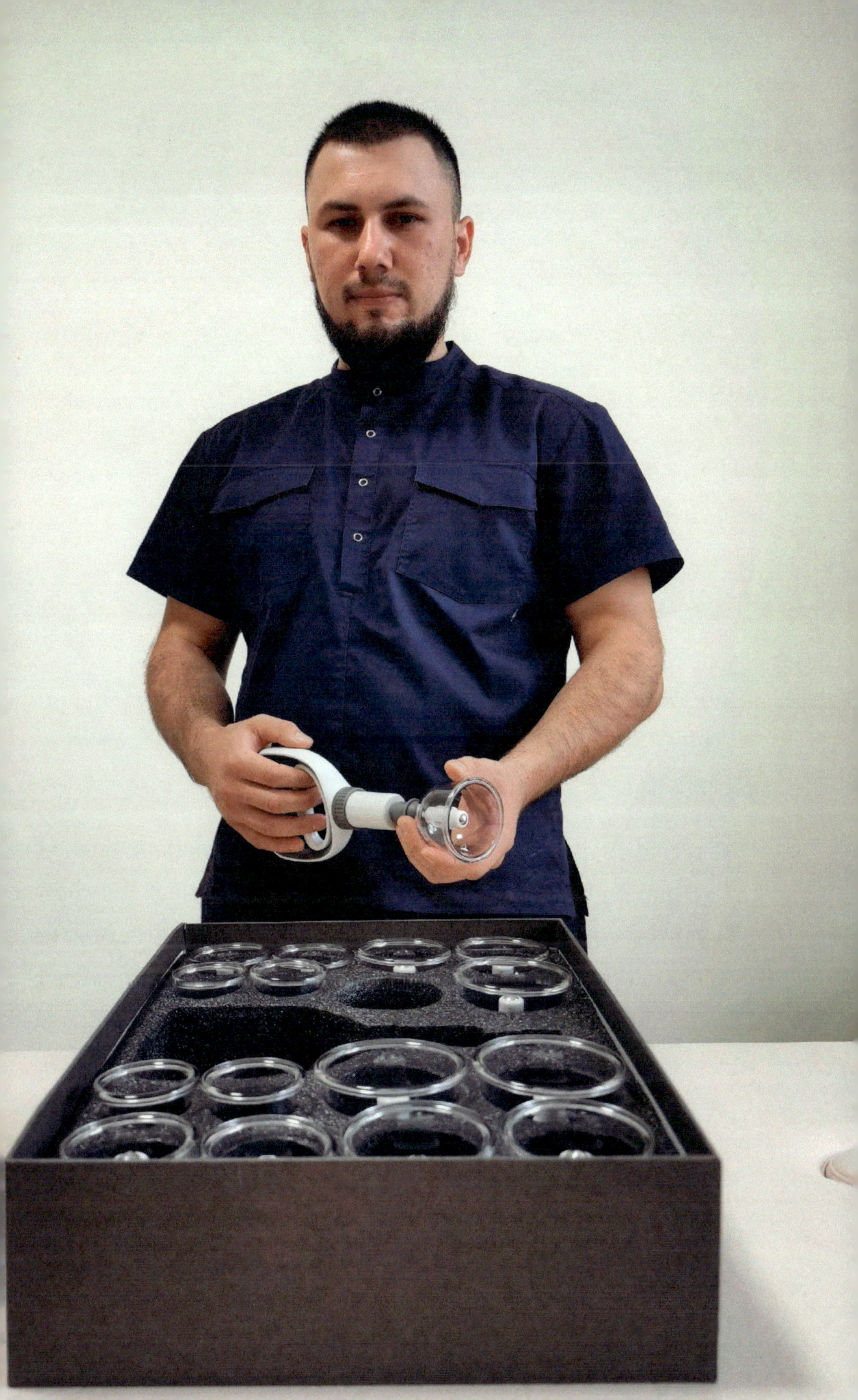

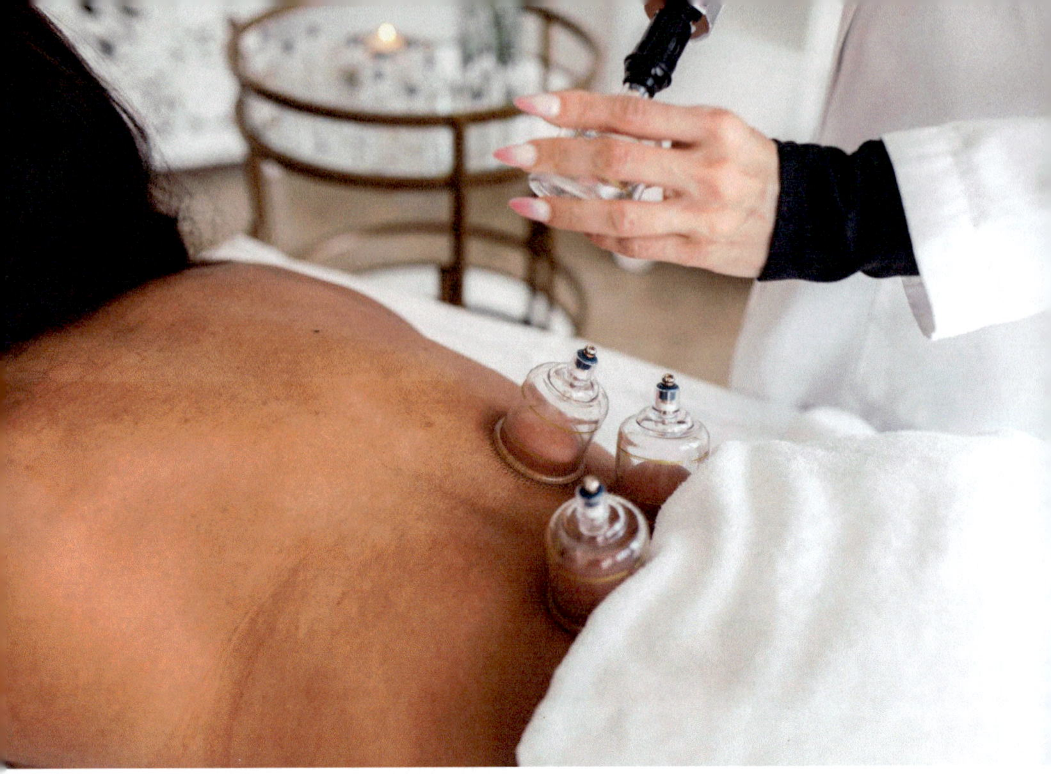

How to Perform Hijama Cupping Therapy a Step-by-Step Guide

In this chapter, you will study about the practical sides of Hijama cupping therapy, such as how to select the right cups, how to sterilize and prepare the equipment, how to apply and remove the cups, how to make incisions and extract blood, how to clean and dress the wounds, and how to dispose of the waste. Additionally, you will discover several exclusive tips and techniques for properly and successfully utilizing Hijama cupping therapy. Hijama cupping therapy is an alternative medical technique that uses cups to create suction on the skin in order to balance the body's energy, improve blood flow, and eliminate toxins. Hijama cupping therapy comes in a variety of forms and techniques, including water cupping, herbal cupping, dry cupping, blood cupping, moving cupping, needle cupping, moxa cupping, empty cupping, and full cupping.

How To Set Up Your Equipment And Space For Hijama

Hijama is a trustworthy and hygienic therapy that requires proper materials and space to perform. Before the treatment, you must arrange the materials and area for the Hijama according to certain rules and guidelines. To get your supplies and area ready for your Hijama, consider the following necessary objects and actions:

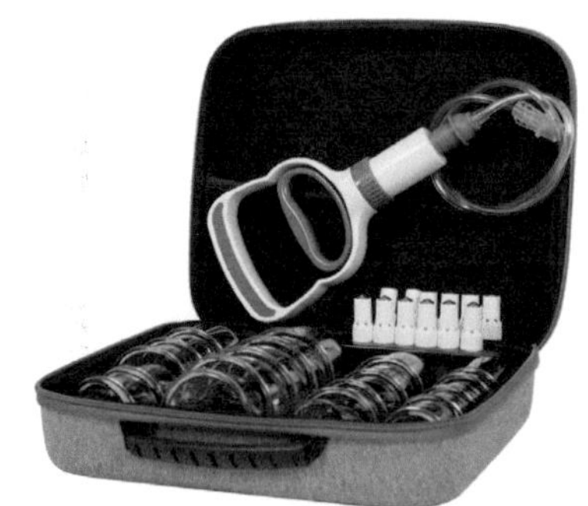

List of Stationary Equipment

You will need some stationary equipment to implement Hijama, such as:

- A bed on which the patient can rest

- A cushion or pillow to support the patient's head or back; a blanket or sheet to cover their body or stay warm

- For the practitioner to see the skin or the incisions properly, a lamp or flashlight

- A timer or clock that allows the practitioner to keep track of how long the Hijama process takes

- A bin or a bag for the practitioner to discard the materials or rubbish

List of Disposable Materials to perform Hijama

To perform Hijama, you will need some disposable materials, such as:

- Cups to help the practitioner establish suction on the skin.

- To produce vacuum in the cups, the practitioner can use fire, manual, or electric methods.

- Razors, needles, or lancets for the practitioner to make incisions in the skin.

- Cotton pads, gauze, or swabs for the practitioner to clean or disinfect the skin or incisions.

- The practitioner can use alcohol, iodine, or hydrogen peroxide to sanitize the skin or instruments.

- The practitioner can apply olive oil, black seed oil, or honey to calm or heal the skin or incisions.

- Plasters, gauze, or tapes for the specialist to cover the skin or the incisions.

Stages to Prepare Your Materials and Space for Hijama

To prepare the materials and area for Hijama, you will need to take the following steps:

- Clean and sterilize your area and equipment before and after each Hijama session.

- Arrange your space and equipment in a pleasant and convenient manner for both you and your patient.

- Before using your materials and gadgets, make sure they are free of faults or damage.

- Use sterile and disposable materials and devices for each Hijama session; do not reuse them.

- After each Hijama session, dispose of your waste and supplies safely and properly.

How to Perform Hijama Cupping Therapy A Step by Step Guide

Ways to Prep Skin for Hijama: Cleansing and Moisturizing

Using vacuum pressure, the Hijama draws blood toward the skin, eliminating pollutants and poisons from the surrounding tissues. Numerous medical ailments, including varicose veins, migraines, back pain, and blood disorders, can be helped by it. It is crucial to appropriately prepare the skin before, during, and after the Hijama process in order to execute it safely and successfully. The actions to take are as follows:

Using Hydrogen Peroxide to Clean the Skin

We use hydrogen peroxide, a chemical substance with bleaching and disinfecting qualities, to clean the skin before beginning the Hijama operation. Hydrogen peroxide not only reduces inflammation and infection but also aids in clearing the skin's surface of debris, germs, and dead skin cells. Although there are many strengths of hydrogen peroxide, 3% is the most often used for skin applications. We use a cotton ball or gauze pad soaked in a tiny bit of hydrogen peroxide, and we gently massage it over the desired area of skin to wear a hijab. Hydrogen peroxide can irritate and harm the eyes, mouth, and nose, so we try to avoid getting it in these sensitive places. Hydrogen peroxide should also not be applied to open wounds since it might impede healing and leave scars. After allowing the hydrogen peroxide to dry on the skin for a short while, we remove it with a fresh cloth or tissue.

Applying Olive or Black Seed Oil on the Skin

Then we apply a thin layer of olive or black seed oil to the skin, which are natural oils with hydrating, anti-inflammatory, and antimicrobial properties. These oils help to keep the skin moisturized and smooth while also increasing the suction of the cups. Olive oil contains monounsaturated fatty acids, vitamin E, and antioxidants, which protect the skin from oxidative stress and inflammation. Black seed oil is made from Nigella sativa seeds, which have been used in traditional medicine for generations. Black seed oil includes thymoquinone, which has anti-inflammatory, antibacterial, antifungal, and antiviral effects. Using a dropper or spoon, we add a few drops of olive or black seed oil to the skin and spread it evenly with our fingertips. We carefully massage the oil into the skin until it is completely absorbed. We don't use too much oil because it can interfere with the vacuum seal on the cups. After applying the oil, we're ready to put the cups to the skin.

1: Patient Consultation and Consent:

This is the first and most significant stage, as it requires the patient's permission and willingness to enjoy Hijama. The practitioner should explain the benefits, risks, and procedures of Hijama to the patient, and answer any questions or concerns they may have. The patient should sign a consent form that states they understand and accept the terms and conditions of Hijama.

2: Filling medical history form:

The second phase entails gathering pertinent data regarding the health and medical background of the patient. Inquiries on the patient's previous and present medical history, prescription drugs, allergies, surgeries, injuries, and lifestyle choices should be made by the practitioner. Along with checking vital signs like blood pressure, pulse, temperature, and oxygen saturation, the practitioner should also assess the patient's health. In order to document the patient's information and observations, the physician must complete a medical history form.

3: Cup Configuration Determination:

This is the third phase, and it entails determining how many cups to use for the Hijama. The number of cups used is determined by the patient's intent and condition, as well as the practitioner's preferences and experience. In general, use fewer cups for preventive Hijama and more cups for curative Hijama. The average amount of cups is four to twelve, but this can vary depending on the scenario. The practitioner should determine the number of cups that are appropriate and safe for the patient. Tailor the Hijama cups to the client's specific needs. Consider multiple factors:

- **Screening Hijama:** Identifying general spots of concern.

- **Aching Areas:** Locating pain points or discomfort expressed by the client.

- **Anatomy Consideration:** Incorporating anatomical knowledge post-health assessment.

- **Nervous System Analysis:** Identifying points related to the nervous system.

- **Diagnosis Methods:** Integrating diagnostic tools for a precise approach.

4: Selecting the cup locations

This is the fourth phase, and it involves deciding where to position the cups on the patient's body. The cup positions are determined by the type and method of Hijama used, as well as the patient's diagnosis and symptoms. There are various methods for selecting the cup positions, such as:

- **Location selection is based on Hijama screening.** This procedure involves scanning the patient's body with a specific instrument or manually identifying the spots that require Hijama. The equipment or procedure detects the electrical resistance or skin temperature of the body and identifies locations with low or high readings. These places are then labeled as cup locations, indicating imbalances or blockages in the body's energy flow.

- **Location selection is based on the painful areas.** This is a strategy that uses the patient's feedback and the practitioner's observation to identify the places that generate pain or discomfort for the patient. The patient is asked to point out or describe the regions that hurt or concern them, and the practitioner examines and palpates the affected areas to confirm the discomfort or condition. These spots are then labeled as cup sites, indicating inflammation or congestion in the body's tissues.

- **After filling out the medical history form, select a location based on anatomy.** This is a technique that employs the patient's medical history and the practitioner's knowledge to identify the areas that correlate to the organs or systems impacted by the patient's ailment. The practitioner analyzes the patient's medical history form and determines the organs or the systems that are affected or damaged by the patient's sickness or disorder. These organs or systems are then mapped to the body's surface, and the areas that correspond to them are designated as cup sites, representing dysfunction or sickness in the organs or systems.

- **Location selection is based on the neurological system.** This is a technique that employs the patient's nervous system and the practitioner's skill to identify locations that are linked to the patient's nerves or reflexes. The practitioner stimulates or tests the patient's nerves or reflexes, such as the spinal nerves, cranial nerves, or meridian points, and then evaluates their response or reaction. The cup placements symbolize the disturbance or weakness in the body's neurological system.

- **Location selection using diagnostic procedures.** This is a technique that employs the patient's diagnosis and the practitioner's expertise to identify areas linked to the patient's diagnosis or treatment. The practitioner assesses the patient's ailment using a variety of methods, including blood tests, urine tests, x-rays, ultrasounds, and MRIs, and then selects the best treatment or prescription for the patient. The cup placements reflect the indication or improvement for the body's healing process.

5: Initial vacuuming

This is the fifth phase, which involves placing the cups on the skin and creating a suction to suck the skin and underlying tissues into the cups. The initial vacuuming is performed without creating any incisions in the skin and serves to prepare the skin and tissues for the following stage. The initial vacuuming can be done using several approaches, such as:

- **Fire cupping.** This approach involves using fire to generate a vacuum in the cups. The practitioner soaks 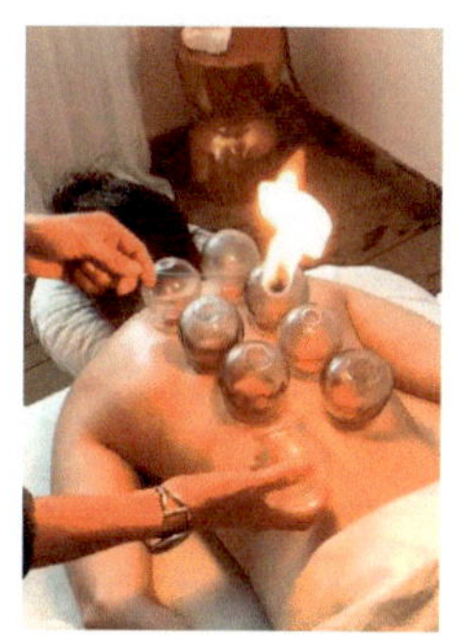 a cotton ball or piece of cloth in alcohol, ignites it on fire, and momentarily inserts it into the cup. The fire consumes the oxygen inside the cup, resulting in a vacuum. The practitioner then swiftly sets the cup on the skin, and the vacuum draws the skin and tissues into the cup. The practitioner repeats the technique with each cup until all of them are on the skin.

- **Manual cupping.** This approach employs a pump or valve to create a vacuum in the cups. The practitioner adds a pump or valve to the cup and squeezes or twists it to remove the air, resulting in a vacuum. The practitioner then places the cup on the skin, and the vacuum draws the skin and tissues into the cup. The practitioner repeats the technique with each cup until all of them are on the skin.

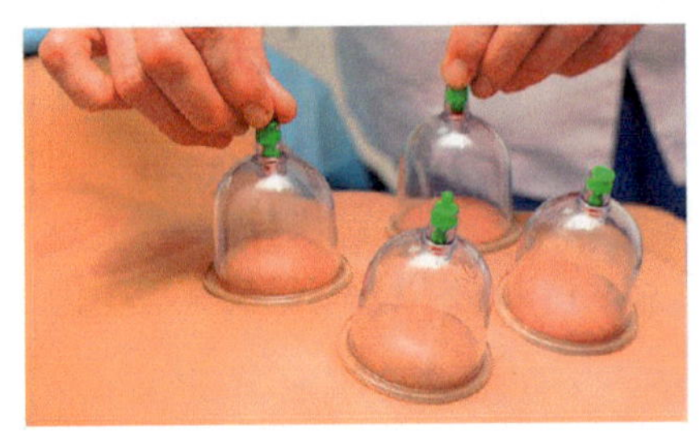

- **Electric cupping.** This approach use an electric gadget to generate a vacuum in the cups. The practitioner connects the cups to an electric device, such as a machine or a battery, and activates it to generate suction, resulting in a vacuum.

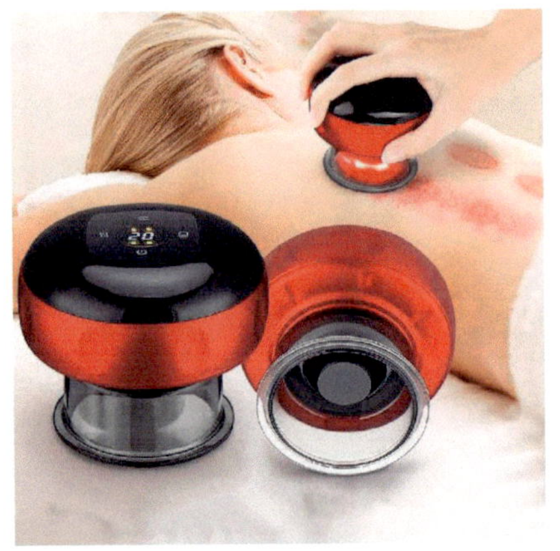

The practitioner then places the cup on the skin, and the vacuum draws the skin and tissues into the cup. The practitioner repeats the technique with each cup until all of them are on the skin.

The initial vacuuming normally lasts 5 to 10 minutes, depending on the condition and the practitioner's preference. The initial vacuuming helps to relax the skin and tissues, enhance blood flow and oxygen delivery, and activate nerve endings and acupuncture points.

Modifying the pressure, duration, and frequency of the cups

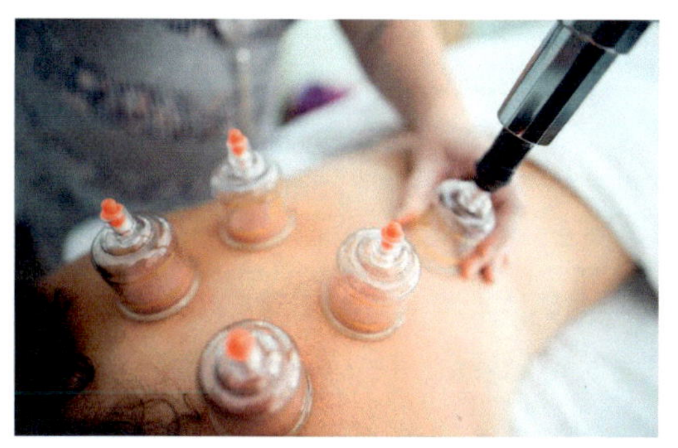

The fourth stage in applying the cups is to modify their pressure, duration, and frequency. The cups' pressure, duration, and frequency govern the intensity and duration of the suction and stimulation, respectively. The cups' pressure, duration, and frequency should be changed dependent on the patient and their health, and this should be done gradually and cautiously to minimize any harm or damage. To regulate the pressure, duration, and frequency of the cups, follow these guidelines:

- Begin with low pressure, short time, and low frequency, gradually increasing them until you reach the optimal level that will generate the finest effects and provide the most comfort for you.

- Monitor the patient's response and reaction to the condition, and alter the pressure, duration, and frequency of the cups accordingly, to obtain the intended impact and outcome while avoiding any negative effects or consequences.

- Experiment with varied amounts of pressure, duration, and frequency of the cups to find the optimal combination that meets your requirements and preferences.

6: Disinfection

This is the sixth stage, which entails cleaning and sanitizing the skin and tools prior to making any incisions. The cleaning is performed to avoid infections or problems after the Hijama surgery. Disinfection can be done using a variety of methods, including:

- **Alcohol.** This approach employs alcohol to disinfect the skin and instruments. The practitioner cleans the skin with an alcohol-soaked cotton pad or gauze, then he massages or dips the equipment. The alcohol eliminates germs and bacteria on the skin and instruments, then evaporates swiftly, leaving no behind.

- **Iodine.** This approach employs iodine to disinfect the skin and instruments. The practitioner applies iodine to the skin using a cotton swab or brush, then soaks or sprays the equipment. Iodine kills germs and bacteria on the skin and instruments, then dries quickly to leave a brown stain.

- **Hydrogen peroxide.** This approach employs hydrogen peroxide to disinfect the skin and instruments. The practitioner sprays hydrogen peroxide on the skin and either rinses or soaks the tools in it. Hydrogen peroxide eliminates germs and bacteria on the skin and instruments, then bubbles up, leaving no stain.

Disinfection often lasts a few seconds or minutes, depending on the type and amount of disinfectant used. The disinfecting prepares the skin and instruments for the next stage.

7: Cutting process

This is the seventh phase, which entails making small, shallow incisions on the skin where the cups will be put. The cutting is done to let blood and poisons to leave the body through the wounds. Cutting can be done with several tools, such as:

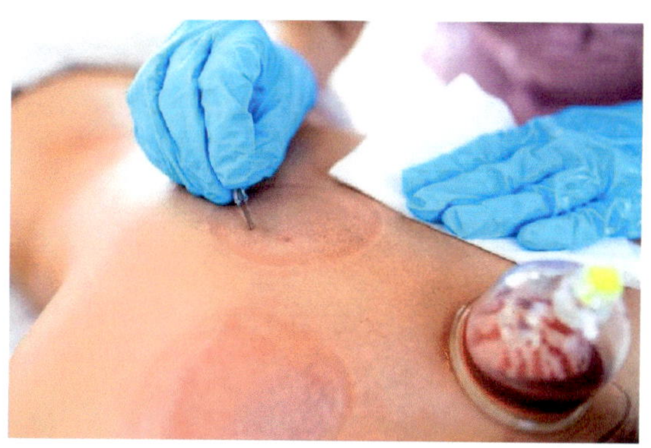

- **Razor.** This is a tool for making incisions using a sharp, thin blade. The practitioner uses one hand to carefully slide the razor over the skin, making small, shallow cuts. The practitioner repeats the procedure for each cup until all of them have cuts under them.

- **Needle.** This is a tool that makes incisions with a pointed, thin metal. The practitioner uses one hand to precisely pierce the skin, creating small, shallow holes.

The practitioner repeats the technique for each cup, until all of them have holes under them.

- **Lancet.** This is a tool for making incisions with a spring-loaded, disposable instrument. The practitioner holds the lancet in one hand and presses it against the skin, creating a small and shallow hole. Following the puncture, the lancet automatically retracts, preventing overuse or harm. The practitioner repeats this method for each cup until all of them are punctured.

The cutting procedure often takes a few seconds or minutes, depending on the tool and the amount of incisions. The cutting technique is utilized to create pathways for blood and poisons to leave the body.

8: Final vacuuming

This is the eighth stage, which entails reapplying the cups to the skin and creating a stronger vacuum to suck the blood and poisons out of the body through the wounds. The last vacuuming occurs after making the skin incisions and is utilized to complete the Hijama therapy. The final vacuuming can be performed using the same techniques as the original vacuuming, such as fire, manual, or electric cupping. The final vacuuming normally lasts 10 to 15 minutes, depending on the condition and the practitioner's preference. The final vacuuming removes blood and poisons from the body and stimulates the healing process.

9: Removing cups

This is the ninth step, which entails removing the cups from the skin and discarding the blood and toxins. The cups are removed when the final vacuuming is completed and are utilized to conclude the Hijama procedure. Cups can be removed via a variety of methods, including:

- **Releasing the suction.** This approach involves using a pump, a valve, or a mechanism to relieve the vacuum in the cups. The practitioner adds a pump, valve, or gadget to the cup and presses or twists it to allow air into the cup, releasing the vacuum. The practitioner then pulls the cup from the skin, allowing blood and toxins to flow out. The practitioner repeats the operation for each cup until they are all removed from the skin.

- **Breaking the seal.** This approach involves breaking the seal between the cup and the skin using a finger or instrument. The practitioner inserts a finger or a tool beneath the edge of the cup and gently pulls it off the skin, breaking the seal. The practitioner then removes the cup from the skin, allowing blood and toxins to flow out. The practitioner repeats the operation for each cup until they are all removed from the skin.

Cup removal often takes a few seconds or minutes, depending on the manner and quantity of cups used. The removing cups is used to remove the skin and tissues from the cups while also disposing of the blood and poisons.

10: Take Care of Your Skin and Incisions After Hijama

Hijama is a therapeutic technique that includes placing cups on particular places on the body to create suction and collect blood and fluids. It is based on the Prophet Muhammad's (SAW) teachings and traditions, which endorsed it as a useful and effective cure for a variety of diseases. To execute hijama safely and efficiently, it is necessary to care for the skin and incisions following the treatment in order to avoid infection and irritation and encourage healing and recovery.

There are several techniques for caring for the skin and incisions after hijama, but one of the most frequent and desired is to forgo bandages and instead use organic substances and appropriate cleanliness. Bandages can be problematic for hijama wearers because they trap heat, moisture, and bacteria, causing perspiration, itching, and irritation. Bandages can also disrupt the natural healing process of the skin and incisions, resulting in scars and markings. Therefore, it is suggested to avoid using bandages for hijama and instead follow these measures.

Cleaning skin and incisions

This procedure involves washing the skin and incisions with a disinfectant such alcohol, iodine, or hydrogen peroxide. These compounds aid in the elimination of germs, bacteria, and viruses from the skin and wounds, as well as the cessation of bleeding and inflammation. To clean the skin and incisions, dip a cotton pad or gauze in disinfectant and carefully wipe away any blood, poisons, or debris. Continue this technique for each cup position until they are all clean and dry.

Applying oil

This stage is applying honey, aloe vera, or olive oil to the skin and incisions. These substances hydrate, feed, and heal the skin and incisions, while also protecting them from infection and irritation. They also contain anti-inflammatory, antibacterial, and antioxidant qualities that complement the advantages of hijab. To apply the ointment or oil, squeeze or distribute a tiny quantity onto the skin and incisions, leaving a thin layer. Massage the ointment or oil gently into the skin and incisions until completely absorbed. Repeat this method for each cup location until the ointment or oil has been thoroughly applied.

Leaving the skin and incisions exposed

This procedure entails leaving the skin and incisions exposed to the air, without any bandages, plasters, gauze, or tape. This allows the skin and incisions to breathe while also promoting natural and rapid healing. It also keeps heat, moisture, and germs from gathering on the skin and incisions, which can cause sweating, irritation, or inflammation. Leaving the skin and incisions exposed decreases the risk of scarring and marking while improving the skin's look and quality. However, this procedure necessitates certain care, such as avoiding exposure to sunlight, heat, cold, water, and chemicals for at least 24 hours after removing the hijama, since these might irritate the skin and incisions and slow the healing process.

Caring for the skin and incisions after hijama is an important and last step in the therapy, determining the treatment's effectiveness and pleasure. By following these measures and avoiding bandages, you can keep your skin and incisions clean, healthy, and attractive, while also making your hijama experience safe, effective, and joyful.

A Comprehensive Guide to Hijama Application: Unlocking the Healing Power

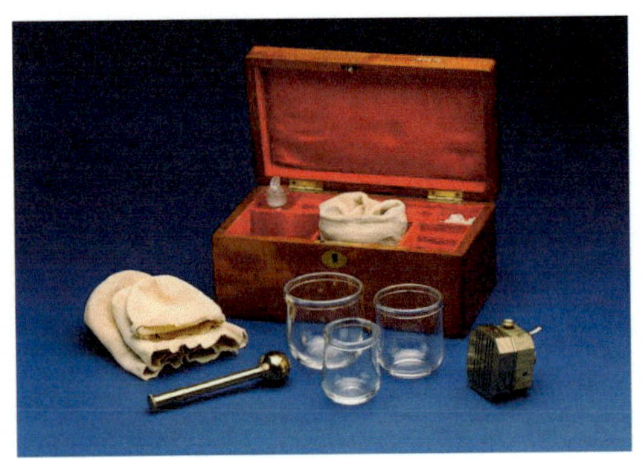

How do you select the appropriate cups for Hijama cupping therapy? How do you determine which cups are best for your needs and preferences? How do you ensure the cups' safety, effectiveness, and comfort? In this chapter, we will address these concerns and more by demonstrating how to choose the best cups for Hijama cupping therapy based on four major criteria: size, shape, material, and quality.

Size

How much suction and how much space the cups can cover depends on their size. When treating a body area or organ, like the back, neck, shoulders, or legs, the size of the cups should correspond with that portion's measurements. Additionally, the size of the cups ought to correspond to the volume of blood or fluids—that is, how much, how little, or none at all—that you wish to remove.

The patient's condition and the size of the cups can determine the diameter, which can vary from 2 to 10 cm. Smaller cups are typically used for areas that are smaller or more delicate, like the face, ears, or wrists, and larger cups are utilized for areas that are larger or more muscular, such the thighs, back, or chest. As opposed to larger cups, which produce more suction and extract more blood or fluids, smaller cups also produce less suction.

The following advice should be taken into account when selecting the appropriate cup size:

- Select cups that will cover the desired area to the fullest extent without going overboard by measuring the area.

- Examine each cup's suction and select the ones that can provide just the right amount of suction—not too much, to prevent discomfort or harm.

- Try on various cup sizes to find the ones that would work best for you and that will also be the most comfortable.

Shape

The cups' design dictates how effectively they fit and seal against the tissues and skin. When treating a certain body part or organ, like the spine, shoulders, arms, or legs, the shape of the cups should correspond with that portion's shape. Additionally, the cups' shape should work with the suction-generating technique—fire, pumps, rubber bulbs, etc.

Depending on the patient and their health, the cups' shapes might range from flat to dome. Generally speaking, flat cups are used for smooth, flat areas like the back, chest, or abdomen, and dome cups are utilized for curved, uneven areas like the elbows, knees, or neck. Additionally, dome cups produce greater suction and stimulation than flat cups do.

The following advice should be taken into account while selecting the appropriate cup shape:

- Examine the shape and feel of the target area before selecting cups that will fit it snugly without being too tight.

- Look for smooth, consistent rims and edges on the cups you select to ensure there are no holes or leaks that could weaken the suction or injure someone.

- Try out several cup shapes, then select the one that will suit you the most and yield the greatest outcomes.

Material

The cup's material determines its durability and safety. The cups should be made of a robust, stable material that is resistant to heat, pressure, and corrosion, like glass, metal, or plastic. The cups' material should also be translucent, clear, or light-colored, allowing for observation and evaluation of the skin and tissues, such as color, texture, and blood flow.

The cups' composition can also influence the manner of creating suction, such as using fire for glass cups, pumps for plastic cups, or rubber bulbs for metal cups. The material of the cups can also influence the patient's and practitioner's sensations and experiences, such as the warmth, weight, and sound.

To choose the proper material for the cups, consider the following suggestions:

- Compare the pros and disadvantages of various materials, such as glass, metal, or plastic, and select the one that best meets your needs and tastes.

- Examine the quality and condition of the cups, and select those that are free of faults, cracks, or leaks, and that can be replaced or fixed if necessary.

- Experiment with different cup materials to see which ones offer the greatest results and provide the most comfort for you.

Quality

The quality of the cups impacts how well they work and how reliable they are. The cups should be of good quality and have been tested and certified by relevant bodies such as the FDA, CE, or ISO. The cups' quality should be constant and assured, and they should be covered by a warranty or a refund policy.

The quality of the cups can have an impact on the outcome and experience of Hijama cupping therapy, including its effectiveness, safety, and patient and practitioner satisfaction. The quality of the cups can also have an impact on Hijama cupping therapy's reputation and credibility because it reflects the practice's professionalism and ethics.

To choosing the proper quality of cups, consider the following tips:

- Check the cups' labels and certificates, and choose cups that have been certified and accredited by the applicable authorities, such as the FDA, CE, or ISO.

- Check the cups' reviews and ratings, and choose the ones with positive and credible feedback from other users and experts.

- Check the cups' warranties and return policies, and select cups with a realistic and fair guarantee and support.

But how do you clean and prepare the equipment for Hijama cupping therapy? How do you ensure that the equipment used for the process is safe and sanitary? How can you prevent infection or disease transmission? In this chapter, we will address these questions and more by demonstrating how to disinfect and prepare equipment for Hijama cupping therapy using various procedures such as boiling, autoclaving, alcohol, and so on.

Cleaning and marking the skin for Cup

The second step in applying the cups is to clean and mark the skin. The skin is the surface on which the cups are put and where suction and stimulation are performed. The skin should be clean and dry to ensure the procedure's safety and hygiene, as well as to avoid infection or disease transfer. The skin should also be marked with acupoints or body parts to ensure the procedure's accuracy and uniformity, as well as to avoid errors or discrepancies.

To clean and mark the skin, take the following steps:

- Wipe the skin gently and thoroughly with a clean, moist cloth or cotton pad to remove any dirt, oil, or sweat that may be present and interfere with the suction or stimulation of the cups.

- Use a clean and dry cloth or paper towel to gently and softly massage the skin to ensure that it is fully dry and that there is no moisture or residue on the skin that could interfere with the suction or stimulation of the cups.

- Mark the acupoints or parts of the body on the skin with a marker or a pen, either using the previous marks or a new source of information, such as a book, a chart, or a website, that provides the names, positions, and functions of the acupoints or areas of the body.

Sterilizing the equipment

Sterilization of equipment is the process of destroying or eradicating any microorganisms, such as bacteria, viruses, or fungi, that may be present on the equipment and cause harm or sickness to the patient or practitioner. Sterilizing the equipment is critical for the safety and hygiene of Hijama cupping therapy and should be done before and after each session. Sterilization of equipment can be accomplished using a variety of methods, depending on the kind and material. Some of the common ways include:

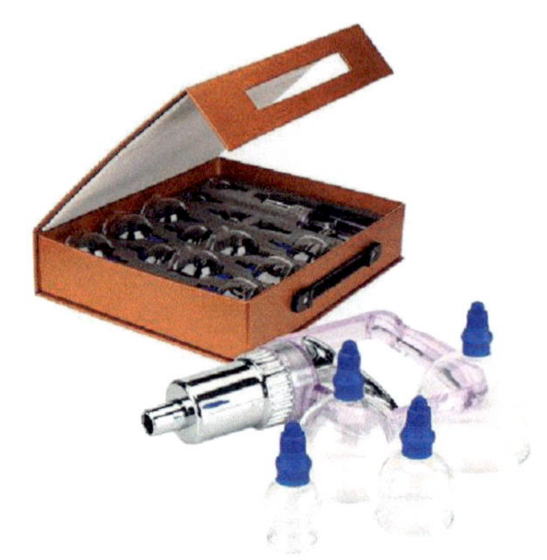

- Boiling: This procedure requires soaking the equipment in boiling water for at least 15 minutes before allowing it to completely dry. This procedure is appropriate for metal or glass cups, pumps, or blades, but not for plastic or rubber cups, as they may melt or deform.

- Autoclaving: Autoclaving is a method of killing microorganisms by placing the equipment in a sealed chamber and using high-pressure steam. This procedure works for metal, glass, or plastic cups, pumps, or blades, but not for rubber cups, which can lose their elasticity or shape.

- Alcohol: This procedure involves soaking or wiping the equipment in alcohol, such as ethanol or isopropyl alcohol, for at least 10 minutes before allowing it to dry fully. This approach is appropriate for metal, glass, plastic, or rubber cups, pumps, or blades, but not for cotton or other organic materials that may absorb or react with the alcohol.

To sterilize the material, you should follow these tips:

- Gather all of the equipment that has to be sterilized, such as cups, pumps, and blades, and inspect it for amount, quality, and condition.

- Choose the right technique of sterilization for the kind and substance of the equipment, such as boiling, autoclaving, or alcohol, and gather the necessary supplies and tools, such as water, fire, steam, alcohol, and so on.

- Perform the sterilization procedure according to the instructions and guidelines, ensuring that the equipment is fully exposed and immersed in the sterilizing agent, and that the temperature, pressure, and time are appropriate and constant.

- Remove the equipment from the sterilizing agent and allow it to air dry fully, or gently wipe it down with a clean, dry cloth or paper towel.

- Store the equipment in a dry, clean, and sealed container, such as a plastic bag, box, or jar, and label it clearly and appropriately, including the date, method, and duration of sterilization.

Observing and examining the color, quantity, and quality of the blood

Examining and evaluating the blood's color, amount, and quality is the third phase in the blood extraction process. The indications or measurements of the blood and the toxins that are extracted, and how they relate to the patient's state and constitution, are the blood's color, quantity, and quality. To evaluate and record the outcomes of blood cupping, as well as to provide feedback and proof of blood cupping, it is necessary to observe and analyze the blood's color, amount, and quality. You should use the following recommendations to examine and assess the blood's color, amount, and quality:

- Discover the type and severity of imbalances or disorders that blood cupping can correct or treat by applying the concepts and theories of traditional Chinese medicine, such as the meridians, the organs, the systems, and the elements, to interpret and comprehend the color, quantity, and quality of the blood.

- Use your eyes, nose, tongue, or microscope, among other observational and analytical tools, to examine and assess the color, quantity, and quality of the blood.

You can also provide data and statistics about blood cupping and demonstrate the patient's progress and condition.

- Utilize books, journals, and websites as sources and references for observation and analysis in order to verify and validate the blood's color, quantity, and quality. You can also present research and evidence supporting blood cupping and demonstrate the legitimacy and dependability of the practice.

Some instances of the color, quantity, and quality of the blood that can be observed and analyzed are:

Bright red blood

This suggests that the patient has strong heart and excellent circulation in addition to fresh, oxygenated blood. Additionally, this suggests that the patient has a yang or heat condition (inflammation, fever, or hypertension), for which blood cupping is a useful modality for calming and cooling the patient.

Dark red blood

This suggests that the patient has weak heart and poor circulation in addition to the blood being old and deoxygenated.

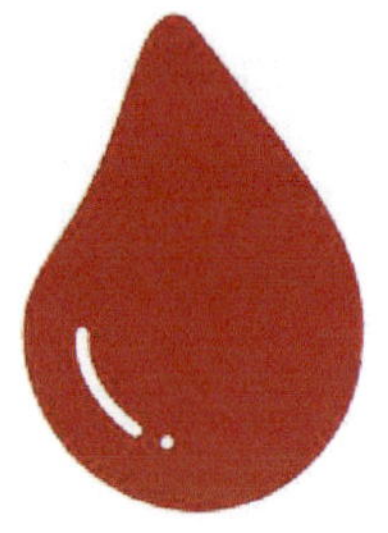

Additionally, this suggests that the patient is suffering from a yin or cold state, such as pain, depression, or stagnation, and that blood cupping can energize and warm the patient.

Thick blood

This suggests that the patient has a high level of waste products and toxins in their blood as well as viscous, sticky blood. Additionally, this suggests that the patient suffers from a moist or phlegm

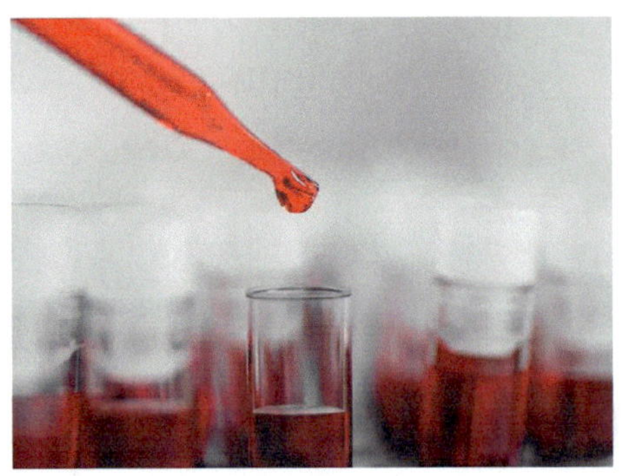

condition—such as obesity, asthma, or edema—and that blood cupping can help the patient clear and drain.

Thin blood

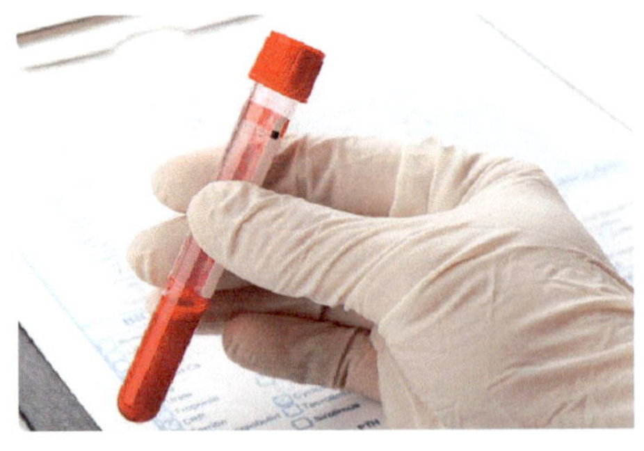

This suggests that the patient has low levels of nutrients and hormones in their blood as well as that their blood is diluted and watery. Additionally, this suggests that the patient suffers from a dry or blood-deficient condition—such as anemia, exhaustion, or insomnia—and that blood cupping can help the patient feel better.

Clotted blood

This suggests that there is a high degree of inflammation and damage in the patient's blood, as well as that the blood has

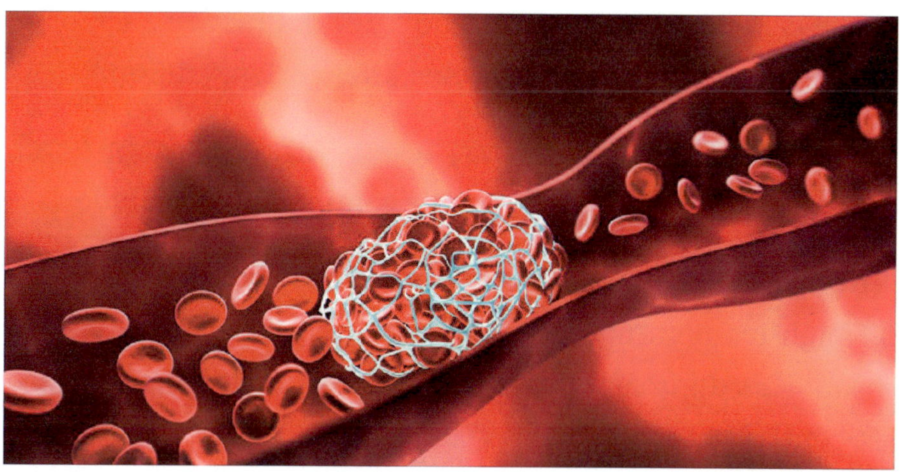

coagulated and solidified. This suggests that the patient may benefit from blood cupping to help disperse and treat any blood stasis or trauma condition, such as bruises, wounds, or scars.

The patient's condition and the amount of blood removed determine how much is taken; typically, 10 to 50 milliliters per cup are taken. The quality of the blood that is extracted is determined by the patient's constitution, but it typically indicates how the body's fluids, blood, and qi are balanced or out of balance. You can assess and record the outcomes of blood cupping, as well as offer comments and proof of blood cupping, by looking at and evaluating the blood's color, amount, and quality.

Disposing of the waste

Disposing of waste is the process of eliminating waste generated by Hijama cupping therapy that may pose a concern to one's health or the environment. Disposing of trash is critical for the safety and hygiene of Hijama cupping therapy and should be completed after each operation.

trash disposal procedures vary depending on the nature and material of the trash. Some of the common ways include:

Incineration: This method involves burning garbage at high temperatures until it is reduced to ashes, gases, or heat. This approach is appropriate for organic, flammable, or contagious trash, such as blood, fluids, debris, cotton, and antiseptic.

Landfill: In this procedure, waste is buried in a defined area and covered with dirt, clay, or plastic. This procedure is appropriate for waste that is inorganic, non-combustible, or non-infectious, such as cups, pumps, blades, and other materials or instruments.

Recycling: Recycling involves reusing or transforming waste into new products or materials while conserving resources, energy, and money. This method is appropriate for waste that is reusable, recyclable, or valuable, such as metal, glass, plastic, or rubber.

To dispose of the waste, you should follow these phases:

- Collect all trash that must be disposed of, including blood, fluids, debris, cups, pumps, blades, antiseptic, cotton, and other materials or tools, and inspect their quantity, quality, and condition.

- Choose an acceptable method of disposal for the waste type and material, such as incineration, landfill, or recycling, then gather the relevant materials and tools, such as a bin, bag, or box.

- Perform the method of disposal in accordance with the instructions and guidelines, and ensure that the waste is entirely and securely enclosed, with no leakage or spills that could cause injury or disease to the patient, practitioner, or the environment.

- To avoid confusion or error, label the garbage clearly and correctly, including the date, kind, and source of the waste, as well as the method and site for disposal.

- Transport the waste to the appropriate disposal location, such as a hospital, clinic, or facility, and abide by the facility's laws and regulations, such as fees, hours, and licenses.

Cleaning and disinfecting the surroundings, the equipment, and the practitioner

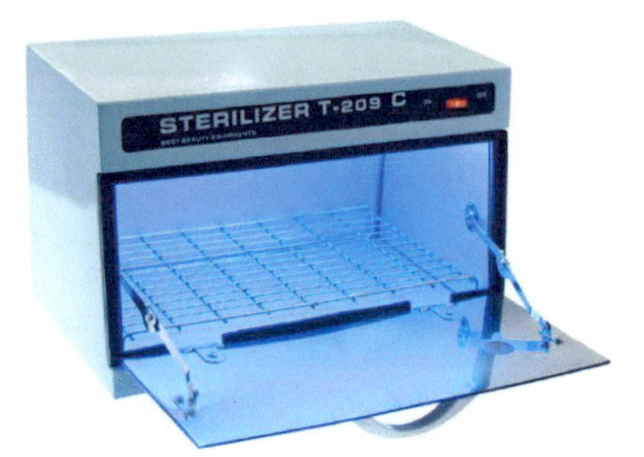

Cleaning and disinfecting the environment, equipment, and practitioner is the procedure of removing any dirt, germs, or residues that may have accumulated on the environment, equipment, or practitioner and may have an impact on the hygiene and safety of Hijama cupping therapy. Cleaning and sanitizing the environment, equipment, and practitioner is critical for the longevity and effectiveness of Hijama cupping therapy, and should be done before and after each operation.

Cleaning and sanitizing the environment, equipment, and practitioner can be accomplished using a variety of methods, including washing, wiping, and spraying. The method of cleaning and sanitizing should be appropriate for the kind and substance of the environment, equipment, or practitioner, such as the floor, table, cups, pumps, blades, antiseptic, cotton, skin, hair, or clothing.

How To Upgrade Your Cupping Equipment Using UV Sterilizers

Cupping equipment, including cups, blades, lancets, and gauze pads, must be disinfected before and after each use to avoid the spread of germs, bacteria, viruses, and illnesses. Sterilization is the process of destroying or eradicating all types of bacteria from an object or surface through physical or chemical means.

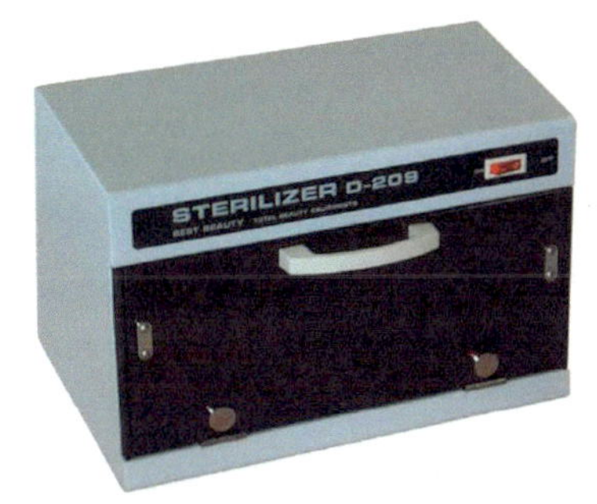

One of the most effective and convenient sterilization procedures is to utilize UV sterilizers, which are machines that employ ultraviolet (UV) light to damage bacteria' DNA and RNA, rendering them harmless and unable to reproduce. UV sterilizers are simple to use, quick, and safe, and require no chemicals or water. They can also increase the longevity and quality of your cupping equipment while saving you time and money in the long run.

If you can afford it, you can acquire a UV sterilizer tool to sterilize your cupping equipment and reap the benefits of this cutting-edge technology. UV sterilizers are available in a variety of models and sizes, both online and at specialist retailers. By buying in a UV sterilizer tool, you can ensure that your cupping equipment is always clean and safe, and that your Hijama sessions are always successful and enjoyable.

The following actions should be taken in order to sterilize and clean the surroundings, the tools, and the practitioner:

- Check the quantity, quality, and condition of all the cleaning and sanitizing supplies and equipment, including water, soap, detergent, bleach, alcohol, cloth, paper towel, sponge, brush, and so on.

- Select a cleaning and sanitizing technique (such as washing, wiping, or spraying) that is suitable for the kind and composition of the surroundings, the tools, or the practitioner. Gather the required supplies and instruments (such as water, soap, detergent, bleach, alcohol, cloth, paper towel, sponge, brush, etc.).

- Follow the directions and guidelines when cleaning and sanitizing the environment, the equipment, or the practitioner. Make sure that everything has been cleaned and sanitized completely and properly, and that nothing remains that could compromise the safety or hygiene of Hijama cupping therapy.

- Make sure the space, the tools, and the practitioner are all fully and naturally dry, free of any moisture or residue that could compromise the safety or hygienic aspects of Hijama cupping therapy. Dry and store all of these items.

Maintaining a high level of hygiene and safety

Maintaining a high standard of hygiene and safety is the process of following the best practices and the precautions that can ensure the hygiene and the safety of Hijama cupping therapy, and that can prevent any infection or transmission of diseases, or any accidents or injuries. Maintaining a high standard of hygiene and safety is essential for the reputation and the credibility of Hijama cupping therapy, and should be done at all times. Ensuring the reputation and legitimacy of Hijama cupping therapy depends on upholding strict standards of sanitation and safety, which need to be maintained consistently.

Here are some pointers to help you maintain a high level of safety and hygiene:

- Use safety gear, such as masks, goggles, aprons, or gloves, to shield the patient and yourself from blood, liquids, or debris exposure. You should also use this gear to prevent accidents, injuries, infections, and the spread of diseases.

- Both before and after the procedure, wash your hands and the patient's skin with water and soap or alcohol to get rid of any perspiration, dirt, or oil and to destroy or stop any germs that could hurt you or the patient, like viruses, bacteria, or fungus.

- In order to prevent any ethical or legal problems, as well as any harm or disease to the environment or public health, dispose of medical waste in a facility such as a hospital, clinic, or other specified location. You should also abide by any local regulations and guidelines regarding this matter, including those regarding fees, hours, and permits.

- To improve your skills and knowledge and to give your patients the best care possible, stay up to date on the most recent research and developments in Hijama cupping therapy. Learn from peers and experts about the advantages, risks, techniques, and equipment.

How to Take Care of Yourself After Hijama?

Hijama therapy is a simple yet effective technique that can have a wide range of health and wellness advantages. However, in order to care for oneself after Hijama, you must follow some measures and suggestions. Here are some of the crucial concerns to consider following Hijama.

Unwind and rest:

After performing Hijama, it's advised to take a few hours to unwind and rest so that the body can repair itself. A Hijama may have a few short-term negative consequences that go away in a few hours or days, like bruising, soreness, or exhaustion. You can lessen these adverse effects and speed up the healing process by getting enough rest and relaxation. At least 24 hours after performing a Hijama, it is advised to refrain from physically demanding activities, exercise, or sexual relations as these can exacerbate blood pressure and heart rate and hinder the healing process.

Eat and drink healthfully:

After Hijama, it is advised to eat and drink enough of water to rehydrate the body and restore vitality. Performing Hijama can result in blood loss, which can dehydrate and weaken the body. Maintaining a healthy diet and drinking habits might aid in the body's fluid and nutritional balance. After Hijama, it's a good idea to sip on lots of water and consume some dates or honey, which can supply natural carbohydrates and minerals. Dairy products, red meat, and processed foods should also be avoided for at least 24 hours after donning a Hijama since they can strain the body's detoxifying and digestive systems.

Clean and treat the wounds:

Cleaning and dressing wounds after Hijama is recommended to prevent infection or complications. Hijama can leave small, shallow cuts on the skin, exposing it to germs and pathogens. Cleaning and treating wounds can help prevent infection and irritation to the skin and incisions. To clean the wounds, use a disinfectant like alcohol, iodine, or hydrogen peroxide, and then apply an ointment like olive oil, black sesame oil, or honey. It is also recommended to cover the wounds with a bandage, such as plaster, gauze, or tape, and change it on a regular basis.

Hijama and Massage

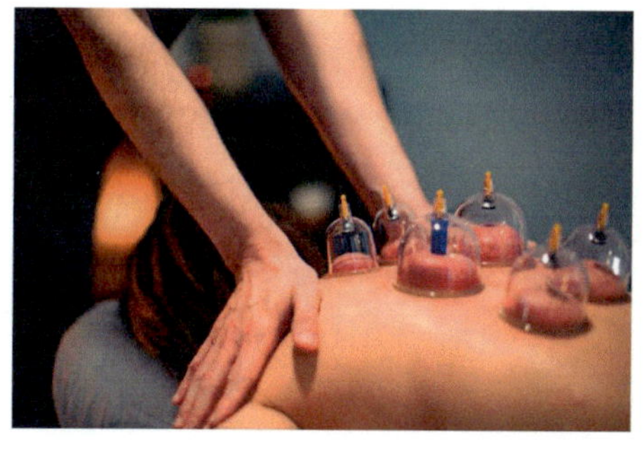

Hijama and massage are two complimentary therapies that can improve your health and wellbeing. Hijama, commonly known as cupping, is an ancient method that uses suction cups to remove stagnant blood and toxins from the body. Massage is a modern technique that combines pressure and movement to relax and activate muscles and tissues. When coupled, Hijama and massage can provide a variety of advantages, including pain reduction, detoxification, relaxation, and stress management.

Pre-Hijama Massage: Prepare for Hijama Cupping Therapy:

- You can prepare your body for Hijama by getting a pre-Hijama massage. This might assist to warm up your muscles and increase blood circulation to the cupped areas. There are two types of pre-Hijama massages to select from, according on your needs and tastes.

- If you are overweight, suffer from joint pain, or have poor blood circulation, a lymphatic drainage massage can help. This is a mild massage that uses small strokes to transport lymph fluid to the lymph nodes, where it can be filtered and emptied. This can help reduce swelling, inflammation, and pain while also improving your immune system.

- A cup massage is appropriate for people with normal blood pressure and circulation. This massage involves gliding a suction cup over your skin to create a vacuum impression. This can assist to relax your muscles, stimulate circulation flow, and gather toxins and pollutants from beneath your skin. This can increase the effectiveness and benefits of your Hijama. Some believe that cup massage can double or quadruple the advantages of Hijama, although there is no scientific proof to back this up.

Massage During Hijama: Boosting the Feeling of Cupping

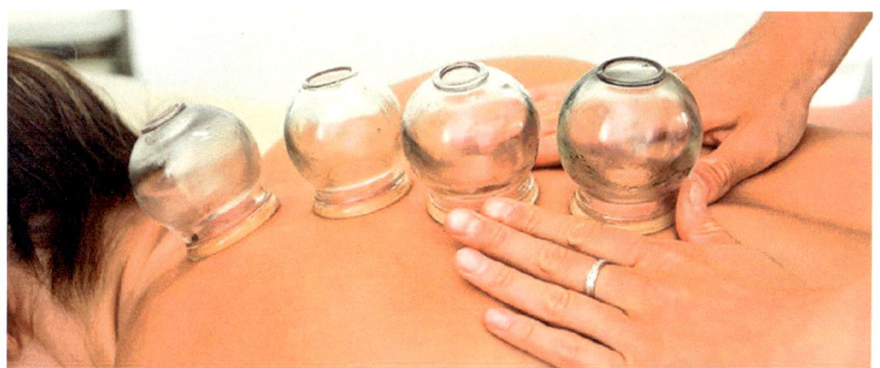

1. Enhancing the cupping experience, while you are having Hijama, you can also enjoy a massage during the process. This can assist to improve the comfort and enjoyment of your Hijama while also increasing its advantages. Depending on the sort of Hijama you have, there are two ways to massage it. Massage the skin before putting the cups might help to loosen and prepare the muscles and tissues for suction. This can also increase blood flow and circulation in the area, boosting the cleansing and healing effects of Hijama. Another option is to massage the skin after removing the cups, which can help to relax the

muscles and tissues and relieve pain or discomfort. This can help increase blood flow and circulation in the area, accelerating recuperation and avoiding problems. Massaging the skin during Hijama helps boost blood flow and circulation in the body, giving you the optimum Hijama results. Massage can also assist to reduce stress, boost mood, and increase overall well-being. Massage while applying Hijama can be an excellent method to improve your cupping experience.

2. If you are using a dry Hijama, which means there are no incisions on the skin, you can use an electric massage tool to massage your legs, arms, or other portions of your body that are not cupped. This can aid to increase blood circulation and oxygen supply to your cells and organs, as well as raise your metabolism and energy.

3. If you've chosen a wet Hijama, which is Hijama with small wounds on the skin to remove blood, you can use a cup massage to massage the cupped area. This can help to enhance suction and pressure, allowing more blood and toxins to leave your body. This can also help to relax your muscles and nerves while releasing endorphins, which are natural pain relievers and mood boosters.

Post-Hijama Massage: Healing and Recovery after Cupping.

- Following Hijama, a post-Hijama massage can help you heal and recover faster. This can help calm your skin and accelerate the healing process. There are two types of post-Hijama massages to select from, according on your needs and interests.

- If you have open wounds from wet Hijama, wait one week for them to heal before having a post-Hijama massage. This can assist to avoid infection or inflammation in the cupped area while also improving your skin's look and texture. You can use oil or no oil, depending on your preferences.

- If you have no wounds from dry Hijama, you can receive a post-Hijama massage immediately soon. This can help to detoxify your body and improve your overall well-being. You can use oil or no oil, depending on your preferences.

Cupping Therapy and Thermal Bath Treatments

Hijama and thermal bath treatments are two natural therapies that can be combined to benefit your health and well-being. Hijama, commonly known as cupping, is an ancient method that employs suction cups to remove stagnant blood and toxins from the body. Thermal bath therapies, also known as balneotherapy, are modern techniques that use hot spring water to calm and invigorate the body. When combined, Hijama and thermal bath treatments can provide a variety of advantages, including pain reduction, detoxification, relaxation, and stress relief.

The Best Time for Hijama and Thermal Bath Therapies:

- Hijama is most appropriate after thermal bath treatments on the third or tenth day. This is because thermal bath treatments can help prepare the body for Hijama by relaxing toxins and impurities that have accumulated in the connective tissue beneath the skin. This can increase the effectiveness and benefits of Hijama.

- If you have Hijama after the third day of thermal bath treatments, you will notice a considerable improvement in your blood quality and circulation. The blood that emerges from Hijama will be darker and dirtier, indicating that it contains more toxins and wastes that are damaging to your health.

- If you have Hijama after the tenth day of thermal bath treatments, you can reap even more benefits because the treatments will have reached their peak length and effectiveness. The typical and optimal spa treatments last ten days, which allows the body to adjust and respond to the thermal bath treatments. The blood that emerges from Hijama will be darker and dirtier, indicating that it contains more toxins and wastes that are damaging to your health.

The Workings of Hijama and Thermal Bath Treatment:

Hijama and thermal bath treatments use distinct but complementary techniques to improve your health and well-being. Hijama works by creating a vacuum effect on the skin's surface, causing the tissue beneath the cup to swell and increasing blood flow to the area. This also stimulates the nerves and boosts the immune system. The vacuum action also draws pollutants and poisons from the skin's deeper layers to the surface, where they are readily removed. This helps to cleanse the blood and lymphatic systems, hence improving overall health.

Thermal bath treatments work by exposing the body to hot spring water, which includes minerals and trace elements that are beneficial to the body. The hot spring water acts as a descaler, penetrating the skin pores and softening the tissues and poisons that have accumulated within them. The hot spring water also relaxes the muscles and joints while improving blood circulation and oxygen delivery to the tissues and organs. This boosts metabolism and energy levels while reducing inflammation and pain.

Reasons to Try Hijama Despite Having Hair on Your Head or Body

Hijama is a strong and natural healing therapy that can boost your health, well-being, and performance. It entails pressing cups against specific points on your body or head to create suction and extract blood and fluids. This helps to cleanse your body of toxins and pollutants while also stimulating blood circulation, the immune system, and energy flow.

However, some people may be hesitant to attempt Hijama because they have hair on their body or head, which they believe may prevent the cups from sticking correctly or cause them pain. They may also be concerned about having to shave their hair, particularly their head, which may not be possible or desirable for a variety of reasons.

If you are one of those persons, we have good news for you: you may still experience the benefits of Hijama without shaving your hair or compromising the treatment's quality. All you need is aqua gel or honey, which are natural ingredients that can assist produce a smooth and sticky surface on your skin, enhancing the suction of the cups.

Aqua gel or honey can also protect your skin from irritation and infection, as well as nourish and mend it after performing Hijama. They are simple to use and remove, and they have no negative side effects. They also align with the Prophet's (SAW) Sunnah, which advised Hijama as a good and effective cure for a variety of diseases.

Chapter
05

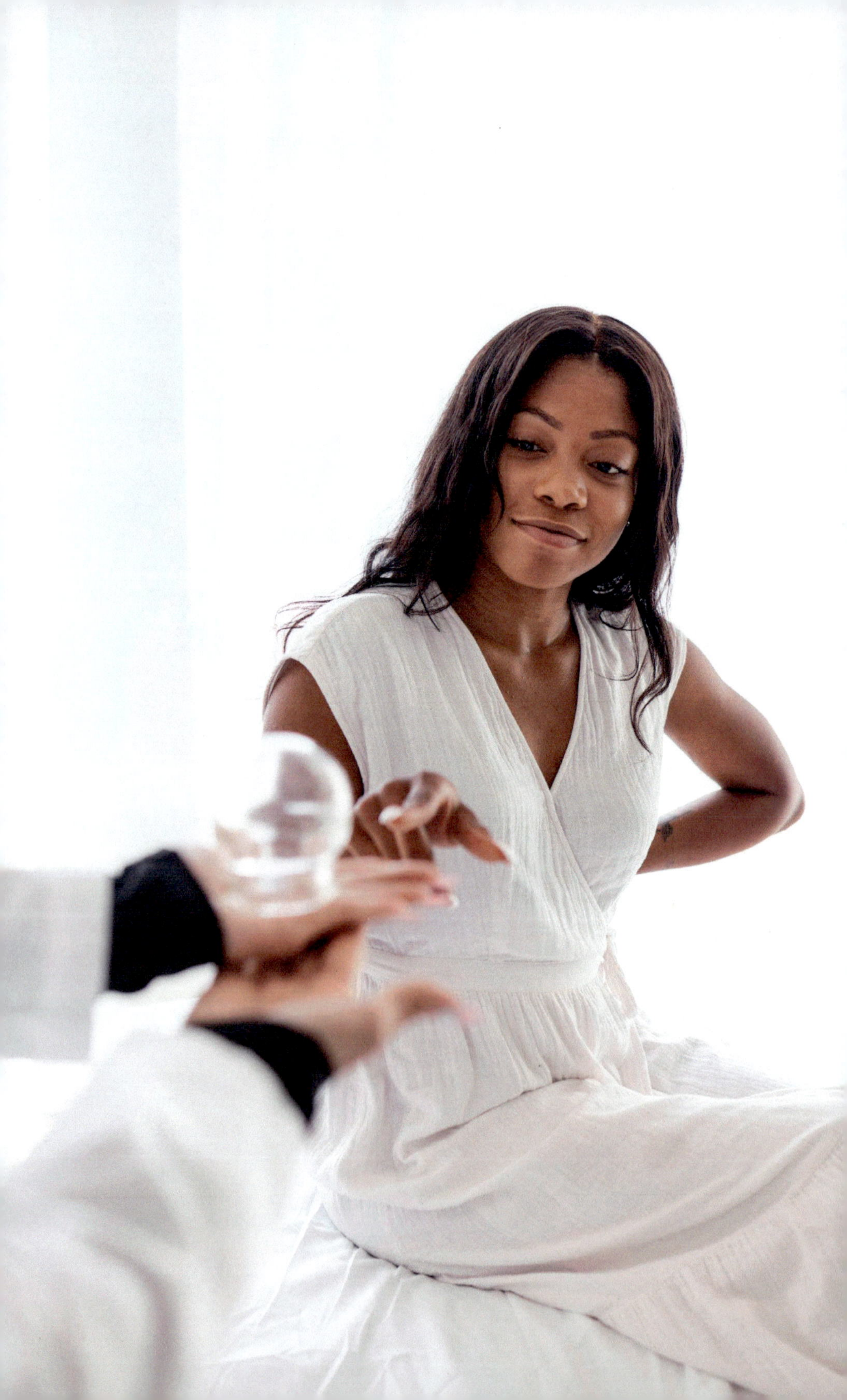

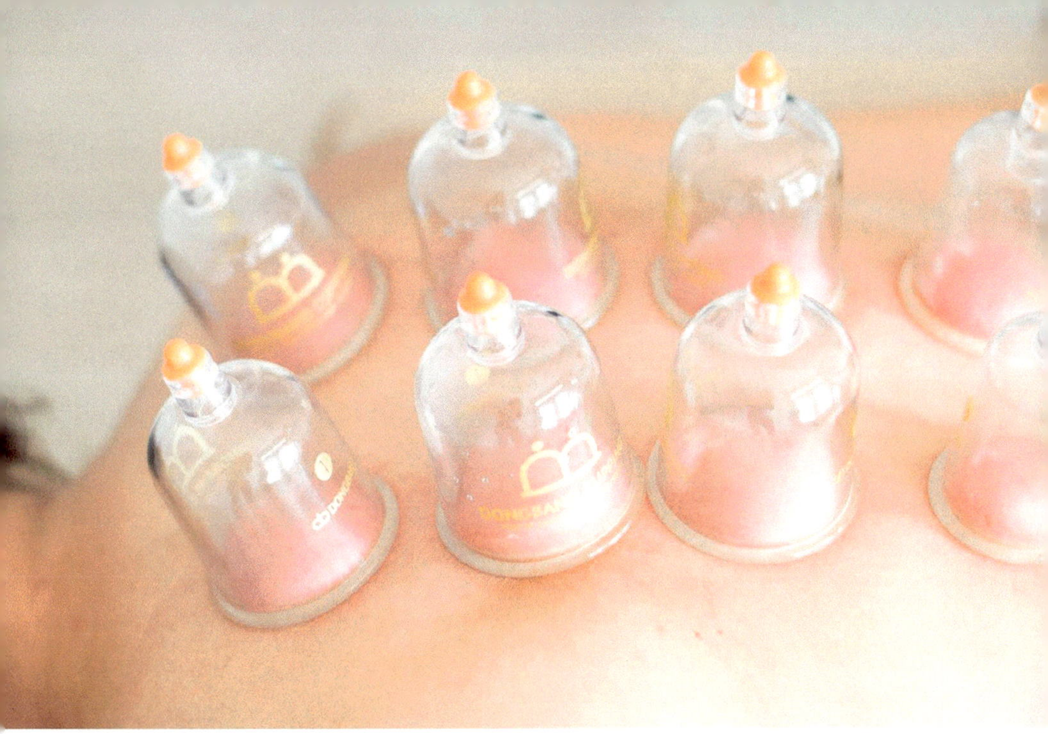

How Does Hijama Cupping Therapy Benefit and Affect the Body, Mind, and Spirit?

Hijama cupping therapy stimulates the neurological system, increases blood circulation, boosts immunity, balances endocrine function, and purges the lymphatic system, among other physiological and psychological benefits.

The production and release of several hormones, enzymes, and neurotransmitters, including endorphins, cortisol, histamine, serotonin, and dopamine, are also influenced by hijama cupping therapy. These factors impact mood, stress level, pain perception, inflammatory response, and sleep quality.

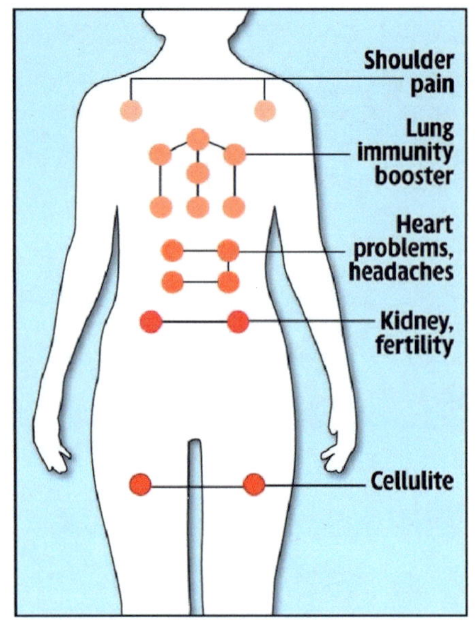

Numerous theories and mechanisms, including the endorphin theory, the gate control theory of pain, the prostaglandin theory, the reflex reaction theory, and the taiba theory, explain how Hijama cupping therapy functions. The therapeutic benefits and effects of Hijama cupping therapy have been demonstrated for a number of illnesses and ailments, including diabetes, pain, hypertension, arthritis, asthma, skin issues, infertility, and more. You will discover more about the benefits and effects of Hijama cupping therapy on the body, mind, and spirit in this chapter.

The evidence behind Hijama cupping therapy's science:

Hijama cupping therapy affects many different bodily systems and functions, which has a multiplicity of consequences on the mind, body, and soul. Following are a few outcomes of Hijama cupping therapy:

Increasing blood flow:

Hijama cupping therapy dilates blood vessels and lowers blood viscosity, increasing blood flow to the area where the cups

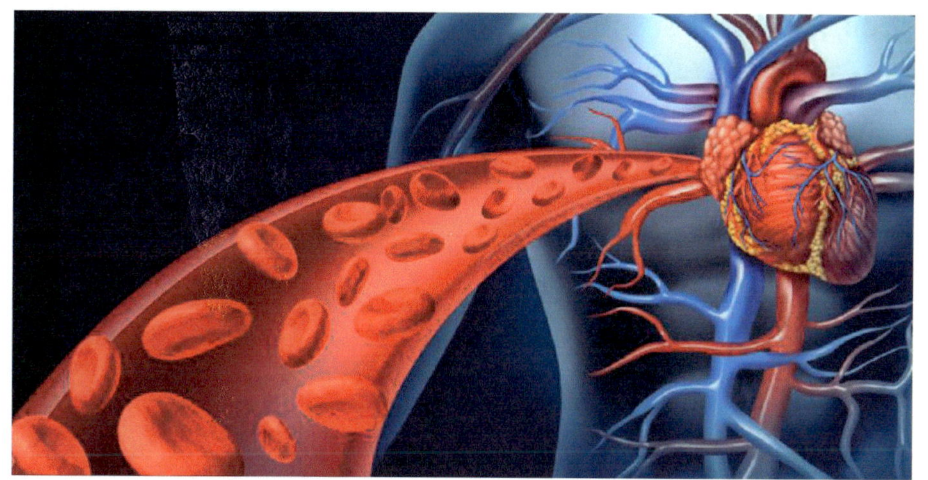

are administered. This accelerates the elimination of waste materials and carbon dioxide and enhances the transport of oxygen and nutrients to the tissues and organs. Because Hijama cupping therapy controls insulin and glucose metabolism, it also helps to maintain blood pressure and blood sugar balance. Because Hijama cupping therapy promotes the synthesis of red blood cells and platelets and inhibits the formation of blood clots, it can also be used to prevent and treat blood problems such anemia, thrombosis, and hemorrhage.

Boosting the immune system:

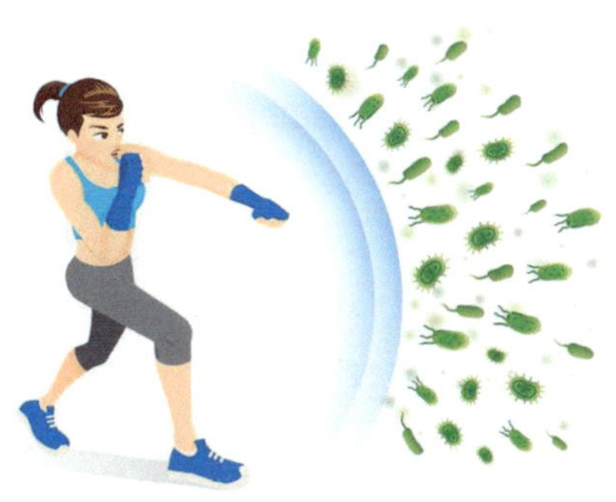

By increasing the generation and activation of several immune cells, including white blood cells, lymphocytes, macrophages, and natural killer cells, Hijama cupping therapy strengthens the immune system. These cells are in charge of fending against illnesses, infections, and foreign objects. Immunoglobulins, which are antibodies that shield the body from pathogens and antigens, such as IgG, IgM, and IgA, are also elevated by Hijama

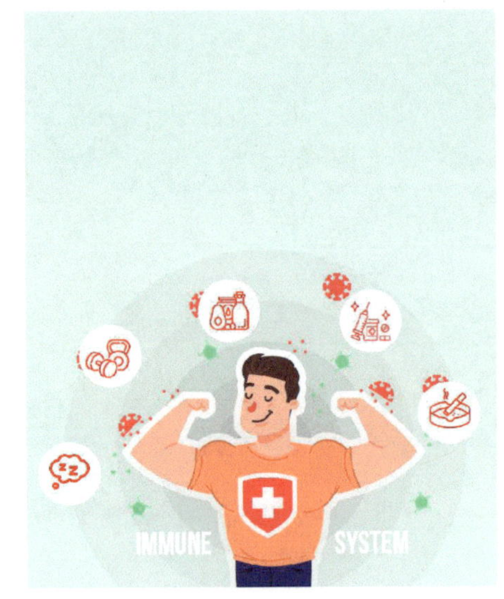

cupping therapy. Because Hijama cupping therapy reduces inflammation and the production of pro-inflammatory cytokines like interleukin-1, interleukin-6, and tumor necrosis factor-alpha, it can also modulate the immune response and prevent autoimmune diseases like rheumatoid arthritis, lupus, and multiple sclerosis.

Turning on the nerve system:

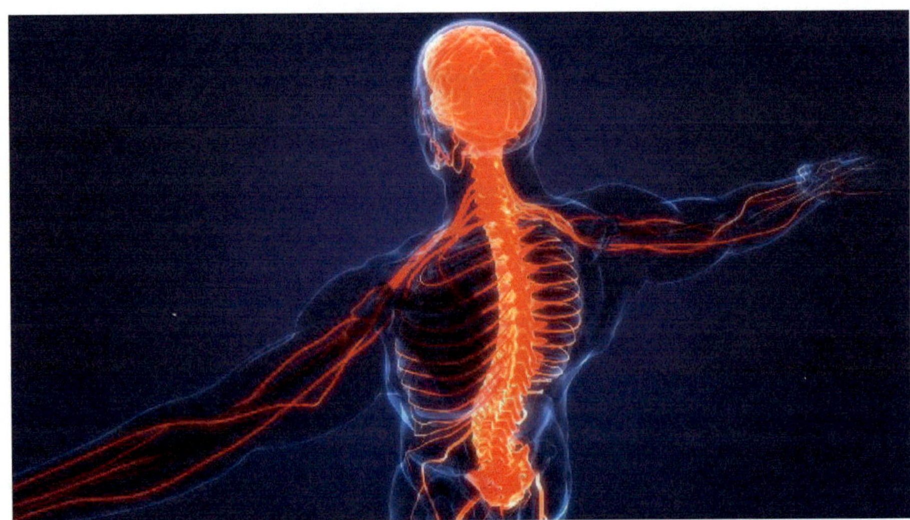

Hijama cupping therapy stimulates the nerve ends and receptors on the skin and muscles, hence initiating the neurological system. This starts the flow of nerve signals to the brain and spinal cord, causing the cerebral cortex, limbic system, hypothalamus, and brainstem to become active, among other parts and processes of the central nervous system. Hijama cupping therapy also affects the peripheral neural system, including the somatic and autonomic nerve systems, and controls both voluntary and involuntary bodily functions, including blood pressure, heart rate, digestion, respiration, and movement. Because Hijama cupping therapy improves blood flow and oxygen supply to the brain and nerves and stops nerve cell deterioration and damage, it can also be used to treat and prevent neurological disorders such as headache, migraine, stroke, epilepsy, Parkinson's disease, and Alzheimer's disease.

Regulating the endocrine system:

By promoting the synthesis and release of several hormones, including endorphins, cortisol, histamine, serotonin, and dopamine, Hijama cupping therapy balances the endocrine system. These hormones affect the body, mind, and soul in a variety of ways, including:

Endorphins: The pituitary and hypothalamus create endorphins, which are endogenous analgesics. They attach themselves to the brain's and spinal cord's opioid receptors to prevent pain signals from being transmitted. Endorphins also lower stress and anxiety levels and produce feelings of euphoria, enjoyment, and relaxation. Hijama cupping therapy provides analgesia and anxiolysis for a variety of pain types, including neuropathic pain, musculoskeletal pain, acute pain, and chronic pain. It also raises endorphin levels in the blood and CSF fluid.

Cortisol: The adrenal glands create cortisol, a steroid hormone. It plays a role in controlling the immune system, metabolism, inflammation, and stress reaction. Cortisol inhibits inflammation and the immune system while raising blood pressure, heart rate, and blood glucose levels. Additionally, cortisol aids in the body's ability to adjust to changes and handle stress. Hijama cupping therapy lowers stress and anxiety levels as well as cortisol levels in the blood and saliva. Because it regulates cortisol secretion and production, Hijama cupping therapy also prevents and treats illnesses of the adrenal glands, including Addison's disease and Cushing's syndrome.

Histamine: Mast cells and basophils both create histamine, a biogenic amine. It plays a role in the control of the immune system, inflammation, allergies, and the release of stomach acid. Itching, swelling, redness, and sneezing are some of the symptoms of allergic reactions brought on by histamine, which also causes an increase in blood flow, vascular permeability, and smooth muscle contraction. Hijama cupping therapy boosts the immune system, reduces inflammation, and raises histamine levels in the blood and skin. Because it controls the synthesis and breakdown of histamine, Hijama cupping therapy also prevents and treats diseases of the histamine metabolism, including mast cell activation syndrome and histamine intolerance.

Serotonin: The brain and the gastrointestinal system both create the neurotransmitter serotonin. It is involved in the control of mood, hunger, sleep patterns, memory, and learning. Serotonin reduces depression, anxiety, and hostility while boosting well-being, happiness, and pleasure. In addition, serotonin controls the circadian rhythm, the sleep cycle, and both the amount and quality of sleep. Hijama cupping therapy enhances mood and sleep quality by raising serotonin levels in the brain and blood. Because it balances serotonin production and reuptake, Hijama cupping therapy also prevents and treats serotonin system illnesses, including depression, anxiety, sleeplessness, and obsessive-compulsive disorder.

Dopamine: The brain and the adrenal glands are the two organs that manufacture this neurotransmitter. It plays a role in the control of movement, motivation, reward, and pleasure. Dopamine reduces fatigue, apathy, and boredom while enhancing creativity, excitement, and enthusiasm. Dopamine also influences balance and coordination, as well as intentional and involuntary movement control. Hijama cupping therapy improves motivation and mobility by raising dopamine levels in the brain and blood. Because Hijama cupping therapy balances the synthesis and degradation of dopamine, it also prevents and treats dopamine system diseases, including addiction, Parkinson's disease, and attention deficit hyperactivity disorder.

Purifying the lymphatic system:

By removing waste materials, toxins, and extra fluid from tissues and organs and transferring them to lymph nodes and blood arteries, Hijama cupping therapy purges the lymphatic system. The lymphatic system is a network of organs, nodes, and vessels that maintains the body's immunity, drainage, and filtration. The lymphatic system also contributes to the preservation of the body's homeostasis and fluid equilibrium. Hijama cupping therapy keeps lymph fluid from building up or stagnating while also enhancing lymphatic evacuation and circulation. In addition to boosting lymphatic immunity, Hijama cupping therapy guards against infections and illnesses.

The physical Advantages and Effects of Hijama cupping therapy

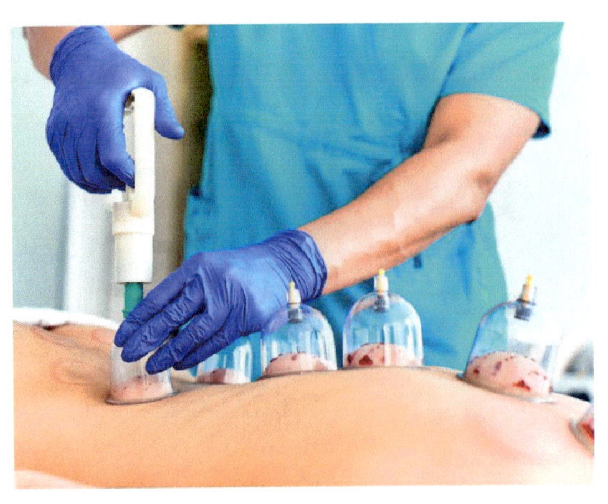

Hijama cupping therapy enhances the health and functionality of the body's many organs and systems, which has a variety of physical consequences and benefits. The following are a few physical outcomes and advantages of Hijama cupping therapy:

The cardiovascular system and the heart

The benefits of Hijama cupping therapy for the circulatory system and heart include:

Increasing blood flow

Hijama cupping therapy dilates blood vessels and lowers blood viscosity, increasing blood flow to the area where the cups are administered. This accelerates the elimination of waste materials and carbon dioxide and enhances the transport of oxygen and nutrients to the heart and other organs. Because Hijama cupping therapy controls insulin and glucose metabolism, it also helps to maintain blood pressure and blood sugar balance.

Treatment and prevention of cardiovascular disorders

Hijama cupping therapy improves blood flow and oxygen supply to the heart and brain, prevents blood clots and plaque from forming in the arteries, and treats and prevents a variety of cardiovascular diseases, including coronary artery disease, angina, myocardial infarction, arrhythmia, heart failure, and stroke. Additionally, Hijama cupping therapy lowers the symptoms and risk factors associated with cardiovascular diseases, including obesity, smoking, high blood pressure, high cholesterol, high blood sugar, and stress.

Improving the liver and the detoxification system

Hijama cupping therapy boosts the health and function of the liver and the detoxification system by:

Cleaning the tissues and blood

Hijama cupping therapy removes waste materials, poisons, toxic chemicals, and extra fluid from the blood and tissues and sends them to the kidneys and liver for excretion. In addition to aiding in the digestion of fats and the removal of toxins, Hijama cupping therapy also increases the synthesis and secretion of bile, a fluid produced by the liver and kept in the gallbladder.

preventing and managing disorders of the liver

Hijama cupping therapy enhances blood flow and oxygen supply to the liver, reduces inflammation and liver cell damage, and prevents and treats a variety of liver disorders, including hepatitis, cirrhosis, fatty liver, and liver cancer. Additionally, the risk factors and symptoms of liver illnesses, including as viral infections, alcoholism, drug misuse, obesity, and jaundice, are decreased by Hijama cupping therapy.

Improving the kidneys and the urinary system

Hijama cupping therapy boosts the health and function of the kidneys and the urinary system by:

Boosting kidney function

Hijama cupping therapy improves renal function by increasing blood flow and oxygen supply to the kidneys. Urine, a fluid that contains waste materials and extra fluid that is eliminated from the body, is produced by the kidneys, which are organs that filter blood. Additionally, the use of Hijama cupping therapy promotes the kidneys' generation and release of renin, an enzyme that controls blood pressure and fluid balance.

Kidney disease treatment and prevention:

Hijama cupping therapy enhances kidney function and stops minerals and salts from building up and crystallizing in the kidneys, which helps prevent and treat a variety of kidney disorders, including kidney stones, kidney infections, renal failure, and kidney cancer. Additionally, Hijama cupping therapy lowers the risk factors and symptoms associated with kidney disorders, including blood in the urine, high blood pressure, high blood sugar, dehydration, and urinary tract infections.

The respiratory system and lungs

The benefits of Hijama cupping therapy for the respiratory system and lungs include:

Enhancing Respiratory Health

Hijama cupping therapy improves lung function by increasing blood flow and oxygen delivery to the lungs. Breathing and gas exchange between the blood and the air, including the exchange of oxygen and carbon dioxide, are functions of the lungs. In addition, histamine—a biogenic amine produced by mast cells and basophils—is stimulated during Hijama cupping therapy. This biogenic amine controls mucus secretion as well as the contraction and relaxation of bronchial smooth muscle.

Treatment and prevention of respiratory conditions:

Because Hijama cupping therapy enhances lung function and reduces lung inflammation and infection, it can be used to prevent and cure a variety of respiratory conditions, including asthma, bronchitis, pneumonia, TB, and lung cancer. Hijama cupping therapy also helps to reduce the risk factors and symptoms of respiratory disorders include allergies, smoking, air pollution, cough, wheeze, shortness of breath, and chest pain.

The gastrointestinal tract and the digestive system

The gastrointestinal tract and digestive system are made healthier and perform better by Hijama cupping therapy because it:

Enhancing the process of digestion and absorption

Hijama cupping therapy improves food digestion and absorption by increasing blood flow and oxygen delivery to the gastrointestinal tract and digestive system. The mouth, the esophagus, the stomach, the small and large intestines, the pancreas, and the spleen are among the organs and tissues that make up the digestive system and gastrointestinal tract, which are in charge of breaking down food and absorbing nutrients. Hijama cupping therapy also promotes the synthesis and release of several hormones and digestive enzymes that aid in food digestion and blood sugar regulation, including insulin, lipase, amylase, pepsin, and gastrin.

Treatment and prevention of digestive problems

Hijama cupping therapy improves food digestion and absorption, reduces inflammation and ulceration of the gastrointestinal tract, and treats and prevents a number of digestive diseases, including gastritis, peptic ulcer, gastroesophageal reflux disease, irritable bowel syndrome, inflammatory bowel disease, and colon cancer. Hijama cupping therapy also lowers the risk of digestive illnesses and their symptoms, including stress, spicy foods, alcohol, helicobacter pylori infection, abdominal pain, bloating, nausea, vomiting, diarrhea, and constipation.

Boosts the reproductive system and the fertility

Hijama cupping therapy boosts the health and function of the reproductive system and the fertility by:

Boosting reproductive function:

Hijama cupping therapy promotes blood flow and oxygen supply to the reproductive system, which improves reproductive function. The reproductive system is made up of a variety of organs and structures, including the ovaries, uterus, fallopian tubes, cervix, vagina, testes, epididymis, vas deferens, prostate, and penis, which are in charge of producing and transporting gametes like eggs and sperm, as well as facilitating fertilization and pregnancy. Hijama cupping therapy additionally promotes the production and release of reproductive hormones such as estrogen, progesterone, testosterone, follicle-stimulating hormone, luteinizing hormone, and human chorionic gonadotropin, which control the menstrual cycle, ovulation, sperm production, and pregnancy.

Preventing and diagnosing reproductive disorders:

Hijama cupping therapy prevents and treats a variety of reproductive diseases, including polycystic ovary syndrome, endometriosis, uterine fibroids, ovarian cysts, pelvic inflammatory disease, erectile dysfunction, prostatitis, and prostate cancer, by improving reproductive function and inhibiting the inflammation and growth of abnormal tissues in the reproductive system. Hijama cupping therapy also helps to minimize the risk factors and symptoms of reproductive illnesses such hormonal imbalance, obesity, diabetes, infections, infertility, irregular periods, heavy bleeding, pelvic discomfort, sexual dysfunction, and urinary issues.

The musculoskeletal system and the joints

Hijama cupping therapy enhances the health and functionality of the musculoskeletal system and joints by:

Strengthening muscle and bone function:

Hijama cupping therapy promotes blood flow and oxygen supply to the muscles and bones, hence improving muscle and bone function. Muscles and bones are tissues that support and move the body while also safeguarding its internal organs. Hijama cupping therapy also increases the creation and release of muscle and bone hormones such as growth hormone, insulin-like growth factor, calcitonin, and parathyroid hormone, all of which govern muscle and bone growth, repair, and metabolism.

Prevention and management of musculoskeletal disorders:

Hijama cupping therapy prevents and treats a variety of musculoskeletal illnesses, including osteoporosis, osteoarthritis, rheumatoid arthritis, gout, fibromyalgia, and muscle spasms, by improving muscle and bone function while also preventing inflammation and bone deterioration. Hijama cupping therapy also decreases the risk factors and symptoms of musculoskeletal illnesses, including aging, menopause, vitamin D insufficiency, calcium deficiency, injury, infection, pain, stiffness, edema, and decreased mobility.

The psychological advantages and effects of Hijama cupping therapy

Hijama cupping therapy includes a variety of mental advantages and impacts, including improved brain and nervous system health. Hijama cupping therapy can have the following mental benefits and effects:

Mood and emotions

Hijama cupping therapy enhances mood and emotions by:

Increasing amounts of neurotransmitters

Hijama cupping therapy increases the creation and release of different neurotransmitters, including serotonin, dopamine, and endorphins, which influence mood, emotions, and behavior. Serotonin improves happiness, satisfaction, and well-being while decreasing depression, anxiety, and violence. Dopamine enhances excitement, enthusiasm, and inventiveness while decreasing boredom, weariness, and indifference. Endorphins cause feelings of exhilaration, enjoyment, and relaxation while also reducing tension and anxiety.

Balancing the cerebral hemispheres

Hijama cupping therapy balances the activity and function of the brain's two hemispheres, each responsible for a separate cognitive process and function. The left hemisphere is related with logic, analysis, language, and mathematics, while the right hemisphere is associated with intuition, creativity, imagination, and art. Hijama cupping therapy improves communication and integration between the two hemispheres, as well as cognitive capacities and skills.

The memory and the learning Ability

Hijama cupping therapy boosts the memory and the learning by:

Increasing blood flow and oxygen availability to the brain

Hijama cupping therapy promotes blood flow and oxygen supply to the brain, hence improving brain function and performance. The brain is an organ that controls and coordinates the body's activities and actions, as well as processes and stores information. Hijama cupping therapy also increases the creation and release of different brain hormones, including growth hormone, insulin-like growth factor, and brain-derived neurotrophic factor, all of which govern brain cell growth, repair, and survival.

The prevention and treatment of neurological diseases

Hijama cupping therapy prevents and treats a variety of neurological disorders, including headaches, migraines, strokes, epilepsy, Parkinson's disease, and Alzheimer's disease, by improving blood flow and oxygen supply to the brain and nerves while also preventing nerve cell degeneration and damage. Hijama cupping therapy also lowers the risk factors and symptoms of neurological illnesses such as high blood pressure, diabetes, smoking, stress, pain, seizures, tremors, and memory loss.

Attention and Concentration

Hijama cupping therapy increases attention and concentration by:

Increasing amounts of neurotransmitters

Hijama cupping therapy enhances the creation and release of several neurotransmitters, including norepinephrine, acetylcholine, and glutamate, which change attention, focus, and alertness levels. Norepinephrine promotes arousal, attentiveness, and focus while decreasing distraction, weariness, and sleepiness. Acetylcholine improves attention, learning, and memory, while decreasing confusion, forgetfulness, and dementia. Glutamate improves cognition, perception, and awareness while reducing impairment, hallucinations, and delusions.

Maintaining Brain Waves

Hijama cupping therapy regulates the frequency and amplitude of brain waves, which are electrical impulses produced by brain cells that represent the state of the brain and consciousness. The brain waves are categorized into five types: alpha, beta, theta, delta, and gamma. Alpha waves are linked to calm, meditation, and creativity. Beta waves are linked to attentiveness, focus, and problem solving. Theta waves are linked to deep relaxation, hypnosis, and dreams. Delta waves are related with profound sleep, healing, and the subconscious. Gamma waves are related with exceptional performance, wisdom, and transcendence. Hijama cupping therapy increases brain wave synchronization and harmony, as well as mental and physical function.

Evidence and demonstrations of Hijama cupping therapy for a range of physical illnesses and ailments

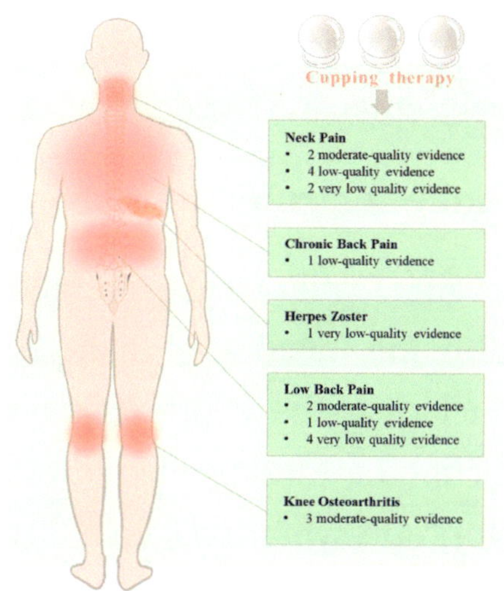

Hijama cupping therapy has been shown to offer therapeutic benefits and effects for a variety of physical ailments and conditions by improving the health and function of different organs and systems in the body. Here are some proof and examples of Hijama cupping therapy for various physical ailments and conditions:

Diabetes

Diabetes is a chronic metabolic illness defined by excessive blood sugar levels caused by an insufficient synthesis or action of insulin, a hormone that regulates blood glucose levels. Diabetes can lead to a variety of problems, including cardiovascular, kidney, nerve, eye, and skin illnesses. Hijama cupping therapy can treat or prevent diabetes through:

Boosting insulin and glucose metabolism:

Hijama cupping therapy enhances insulin and glucose metabolism by boosting blood flow and oxygen delivery to the pancreas, the organ responsible for insulin production and secretion. Hijama cupping therapy also promotes insulin synthesis and release while increasing insulin sensitivity and absorption by cells. Hijama cupping therapy also lowers blood glucose levels, preventing hyperglycemia and hypoglycemia.

Preventing and managing diabetic problems:

Hijama cupping therapy prevents and treats diabetes problems by improving the health and function of diabetes-affected organs and systems, including the heart, kidneys, nerves, eyes, and skin. Hijama cupping therapy also lowers diabetes complications' risk factors and symptoms, including high blood pressure, high cholesterol, high blood sugar, obesity, smoking, stress, discomfort, numbness, tingling, blurred vision, and skin infections.

Here are some instances of Hijama cupping therapy for diabetes:

- Al-Bedah et al. (2019) investigated the efficacy of Hijama cupping therapy on glycemic control and lipid profile in individuals with type 2 diabetes mellitus. The study included 60 patients, who were randomly assigned to either the Hijama or control groups. The Hijama group received Hijama cupping therapy on the back, abdomen, and legs once a week for four weeks, while the control group received no treatment. The results showed that the Hijama group had significantly lower fasting blood glucose, glycosylated hemoglobin, total cholesterol, low-density lipoprotein cholesterol, and triglycerides than the control group. The study found that Hijama cupping therapy improved the glycemic management and lipid profile of patients with type 2 diabetes.

Pain

Pain is an unpleasant sensory and emotional experience that is linked to actual or probable tissue damage, or described as such. Pain is split into two types: acute pain and chronic pain. Acute pain is defined as short-term discomfort induced by an injury, infection, or surgery and lasting less than six months. Chronic pain is defined as pain that lasts or recurs for more than six months and can be caused by a variety of conditions, including arthritis, cancer, fibromyalgia, or neuropathy. Hijama cupping therapy can alleviate or prevent pain by:

Boosting endorphin levels

Hijama cupping therapy raises the amounts of endorphins, which are natural painkillers produced by the pituitary gland and hypothalamus. Endorphins attach to opioid receptors in the brain and spinal cord, inhibiting the transmission of pain signals. Endorphins also produce feelings of euphoria, enjoyment, and relaxation while lowering tension and anxiety levels.

The modulating Pain Perception

Hijama cupping therapy alters pain perception by activating nerve endings and receptors on the skin and muscles, which send signals to the spinal cord and brain, modulating pain perception. Hijama cupping therapy lowers pain intensity and duration by blocking the gate or passage that sends pain signals from peripheral nerves to the central nervous system.

Here are some examples of Hijama cupping therapy for pain:

- Cao et al. (2010) conducted a meta-analysis to assess the effectiveness of Hijama cupping therapy for pain management in a variety of conditions, including low back pain, neck pain, shoulder pain, headache, and knee pain. The meta-analysis included 16 randomized controlled trials that compared Hijama cupping therapy to standard therapies like medicine, acupuncture, massage, and physiotherapy. The findings revealed that Hijama cupping therapy has a substantial effect on pain reduction when compared to conventional treatments. The meta-analysis found that Hijama cupping therapy was an effective treatment for a variety of ailments.

Hypertension

Hypertension is a chronic disorder defined by high blood pressure, which is the force of blood against the walls of the arteries. Hypertension can lead to a variety of consequences, including cardiovascular disorders, renal disease, stroke, and eye disease. Hijama cupping therapy treats or prevents hypertension by:

Enhancing blood circulation

Hijama cupping therapy promotes blood circulation by boosting blood flow to the area where the cups are applied, dilating the blood vessels and decreasing blood viscosity. This reduces the resistance and pressure of the blood against the artery walls, so balancing blood pressure.

Controlling the renin-angiotensin-aldosterone system

Hijama cupping therapy affects the renin-angiotensin-aldosterone system, a hormonal system that controls blood pressure and fluid levels. Hijama cupping therapy stimulates the creation and release of renin, an enzyme produced by the kidneys that converts angiotensinogen, a protein produced by the liver, into angiotensin I, which is then converted into angiotensin II, a powerful vasoconstrictor that raises blood pressure. Hijama cupping therapy also reduces the generation and release of angiotensin-converting enzyme, which converts angiotensin I to angiotensin II. Hijama cupping therapy also lowers the production and release of aldosterone, a hormone produced by the adrenal glands, while increasing the kidneys' reabsorption of sodium and water, which raises blood volume and blood pressure.

Here are some instances of Hijama cupping therapy for hypertension:

- Arslan et al. (2014) investigated the effect of Hijama cupping therapy on the blood pressure and lipid profiles of hypertensive individuals. The study included 40 patients, who were randomly assigned to either the Hijama or control groups. The Hijama group received Hijama cupping therapy on the back, abdomen, and legs once a week for four weeks, while the control group received no treatment. The study found that the Hijama group had significantly lower systolic and diastolic blood pressure, total cholesterol, low-density lipoprotein cholesterol, and triglycerides than the control group. Hijama cupping therapy was found to enhance the blood pressure and lipid profile of hypertensive individuals.

Arthritis

Arthritis is a chronic inflammatory illness of the joints that causes pain, stiffness, swelling, and decreased movement. Arthritis is split into two types: osteoarthritis and rheumatoid arthritis. Osteoarthritis is a degenerative disease that affects both cartilage and bone, producing wear and tear and friction in the joints. Rheumatoid arthritis is an autoimmune illness that affects the synovium and membranes, resulting in joint inflammation and destruction. Hijama cupping therapy can be used to cure or prevent arthritis.

Lowering inflammation and pain

Hijama cupping therapy relieves inflammation and pain by improving blood flow and oxygen delivery to the joints while also removing toxic chemicals, toxins, waste products, and excess fluids from them. Hijama cupping therapy also increases the creation and release of anti-inflammatory and analgesic mediators such as endorphins, cortisol, prostaglandins, and histamine, which regulate inflammation and pain perception.

Preventing and managing joint damage

Hijama cupping therapy prevents and treats joint disease by enhancing the health and function of the cartilage, bone, synovium, and membrane while also reducing joint tissue degradation and damage. Hijama cupping therapy also increases the creation and release of growth and repair hormones such as growth hormone, insulin-like growth factor, and brain-derived neurotrophic factor, all of which regulate joint tissue growth, repair, and survival.

Here are some instances of Hijama cupping therapy for arthritis:

- Lee et al. (2018) conducted a systematic study to assess the effect of Hijama cupping therapy on pain alleviation and quality of life in osteoarthritis patients. The comprehensive analysis included 11 randomized controlled studies that compared Hijama cupping therapy to sham cupping, no treatment, or standard treatments like medicine, acupuncture, massage, and exercise. The findings revealed that Hijama cupping therapy had a substantial impact on pain alleviation and quality of life when compared to other interventions.

The systematic study found that Hijama cupping therapy was both safe and beneficial for osteoarthritis.

Asthma

Asthma is a chronic respiratory illness characterized by difficulties breathing, wheezing, coughing, and chest tightness. Allergies, infections, pollution, stress, and exercise are all potential triggers for asthma. Asthma can result in a variety of consequences, including respiratory failure, pneumonia, and lung damage. Hijama cupping therapy can be used to treat or prevent asthma.

- Improving Lung Function: Hijama cupping therapy enhances lung function by improving blood flow and oxygen delivery to the lungs while also enhancing breathing and gas exchange. Hijama cupping therapy also stimulates the creation and release of different bronchodilators and anti-inflammatory mediators, including histamine, serotonin, and prostaglandins, which regulate bronchial smooth muscle contraction and relaxation, as well as mucus secretion.

- Asthma attacks are prevented and treated with Hijama cupping therapy, which improves the immune system and allergic response while also reducing inflammation and infection of the airways. Hijama cupping therapy also lowers the risk factors and symptoms of asthma attacks, including allergens, viruses, germs, dust, smoke, stress, wheeze, cough, shortness of breath, and chest pain.

Here are some instances of Hijama cupping therapy for asthma:

- Cao et al. (2015) conducted a meta-analysis to assess the efficacy of Hijama cupping therapy on lung function and quality of life in asthma patients. The meta-analysis included 12 randomized controlled trials that compared Hijama cupping therapy to sham cupping, no treatment, or standard treatments such medicine, acupuncture, massage, and inhalation. The findings revealed that Hijama cupping therapy had a substantial impact on lung function and quality of life when compared to other interventions. The meta-analysis found that Hijama cupping therapy was both safe and beneficial for asthma.

Skin issues

Skin disorders include itching, rash, redness, swelling, scaling, cracking, bleeding, and infection. Skin issues can be caused by a variety of factors, including allergies, infections, inflammation, autoimmune illnesses, hormone imbalance, and environmental exposure. Skin disorders can have an impact on a person's look, comfort level, and confidence. Hijama cupping therapy can treat or prevent skin issues through:

- Improving Skin Health and Function: Hijama cupping therapy enhances skin health and function by increasing blood flow and oxygen supply to the skin, as well as improving nutritional and hydration levels. Hijama cupping therapy also stimulates the creation and release of different skin hormones and factors, including collagen, elastin, hyaluronic acid, and growth factor, which govern the structure, elasticity, and regeneration of the skin.

- Preventing and treating skin illnesses and problems. Hijama cupping therapy prevents and treats a variety of skin diseases and disorders, including acne, eczema, psoriasis, dermatitis, herpes, and fungal infections, by improving skin health and function while also preventing inflammation and infection. Hijama cupping therapy also lowers the risk and symptoms of skin diseases and disorders, including stress, hormones, bacteria, viruses, fungi, parasites, itching, rash, redness, swelling, scaling, cracking, bleeding, and infection.

Here are some instances of Hijama cupping therapy for skin issues:

- Al-Hashimi et al. (2017) described the effects of Hijama cupping therapy on a 35-year-old female patient with psoriasis and vitiligo. The patient had psoriasis and vitiligo for ten years, and she had grown areas of red, scaly, and itchy skin, as well as patches of white, depigmented, and dry skin, on various regions of her body, which harmed her self-esteem and standard of living. The patient had Hijama cupping therapy on the afflicted areas twice a week for six weeks, in addition to standard medical care. The results demonstrated that the patient's skin look, color, and texture improved significantly following Hijama cupping therapy. The case study indicated that Hijama cupping therapy effectively treated psoriasis and vitiligo while also improving the patient's skin health and function.

Infertility

Infertility is a condition that impairs the capacity to conceive or bring a pregnancy to term. Infertility can be caused by a number of causes, including hormone imbalance, ovulation disorders, tubal obstruction, uterine abnormalities, sperm abnormalities, and genetic flaws. Infertility can have an impact on a person's physical, mental, emotional, and social health. Hijama cupping therapy can be used to cure or prevent infertility:

- Boosting the reproductive system: Hijama cupping therapy boosts the reproductive system by bringing more blood and oxygen to it. This makes it easier for gametes like eggs and sperm to be made and moved around, which leads to better fertilization and pregnancy. It also increases the production and release of reproductive hormones like estrogen, progesterone, testosterone, follicle-stimulating hormone, luteinizing hormone, and human chorionic gonadotropin. These hormones control the menstrual cycle, ovulation, sperm production, and pregnancy.

- preventing and diagnosing reproductive diseases and disorders: Hijama cupping therapy can help with a number of reproductive diseases and disorders, including polycystic ovary syndrome, endometriosis, uterine fibroids, ovarian cysts, pelvic inflammatory disease, erectile dysfunction, prostatitis, and prostate cancer. This is because it improves reproductive function and stops the growth of abnormal tissues and inflammation in the reproductive system. Not only does Hijama cupping treatment lower the risk of reproductive diseases and disorders, but it also lowers the symptoms of them. These include hormonal imbalances, obesity, diabetes, infections, infertility, irregular periods, heavy bleeding, pelvic pain, sexual dysfunction, and urinary problems.

The implications and spiritual advantages of Hijama cupping therapy

Hijama cupping therapy has a variety of spiritual advantages and impacts since it links and aligns the body, mind, and spirit while also increasing knowledge and consciousness of oneself, others, and the divine. Hijama cupping therapy has several spiritual benefits and consequences, including:

The relationship and alignment of the body, mind, and spirit

Hijama cupping therapy helps to unite and align the body, mind, and spirit by:

Restoring the balance of vital energy, or life force:

Hijama cupping therapy restores the equilibrium of vital energy, or life force, which is the foundation of creation and existence. The vital energy or life force is also known as the ruh, nafs, qi, prana, or chi, depending on the culture and traditions. The vital energy, or life force, travels through the body and soul, ensuring the health and balance of the entire being. Hijama cupping therapy restores the balance of vital energy, or life force, by removing the blockages and disturbances that cause imbalance and disharmony in the body, mind, and spirit.

Improving communication and integration of the body, mind, and spirit

Hijama cupping therapy improves communication and integration of the body, mind, and spirit by stimulating nerve endings and receptors on the skin and muscles, triggering nerve impulse transmission to the brain and spinal cord, and activating various regions and functions of the central nervous system, including the cerebral cortex, limbic system, hypothalamus, and brainstem. Hijama cupping therapy also affects the peripheral neural system, including the autonomic and somatic nervous systems, and regulates the body's involuntary and voluntary functions, such as heart rate, blood pressure, digestion, respiration, and movement.

Hijama cupping therapy also balances the frequency and amplitude of brain waves, which are electrical impulses produced by brain cells and represent the state of the brain and consciousness. Hijama cupping therapy also increases the creation and release of hormones, enzymes, and neurotransmitters such as endorphins, cortisol, histamine, serotonin, and dopamine, all of which influence the body's activities and responses, including pain, inflammation, stress, mood, and sleep.

Hijama cupping therapy also boosts the synthesis and release of immune cells, including white blood cells, lymphocytes, macrophages, and natural killer cells, which fight infections, illnesses, and foreign substances. Hijama cupping therapy also increases the creation and release of growth and repair hormones such as growth hormone, insulin-like growth factor, and brain-derived neurotrophic factor, all of which regulate cell and tissue growth, repair, and survival. Hijama cupping therapy also increases the generation and release of spiritual hormones and components such as ruh, nafs, qi, prana, or chi, which govern the body's balance, harmony, and connection to the spirit.

The awareness and consciousness of oneself, others, and the divine

Hijama cupping therapy raises knowledge and consciousness about oneself, others, and the divine by:

- Increasing neurotransmitter levels: Hijama cupping therapy boosts the levels of neurotransmitters like serotonin, dopamine, and endorphins, which influence mood, emotions, and behavior. Serotonin improves happiness, satisfaction, and well-being while decreasing depression, anxiety, and violence. Dopamine enhances excitement, enthusiasm, and inventiveness while decreasing boredom, weariness, and indifference. Endorphins cause feelings of exhilaration, enjoyment, and relaxation while also reducing tension and anxiety. These neurotransmitters also improve cognitive capacities and skills such as logic, analysis, language, arithmetic, intuition, creativity, imagination, and art, as well as raising knowledge and consciousness of oneself, others, and the divine.

- Hijama cupping therapy balances the activity and function of the brain's two hemispheres, which are responsible for distinct cognitive processes and functions. The left hemisphere is related with logic, analysis, language, and mathematics, whereas the right hemisphere is linked to intuition, creativity, imagination, and art. Hijama cupping therapy improves communication and integration between the two hemispheres, as well as cognitive capacities and skills. Hijama cupping therapy also balances brain waves, which are electrical impulses produced by brain cells and reflect the state of the brain and psyche.

- The brain waves are categorized into five types: alpha, beta, theta, delta, and gamma. Alpha waves are linked to calm, meditation, and creativity. Beta waves are linked to attentiveness, focus, and problem solving.

Theta waves are linked to deep relaxation, hypnosis, and dreams. Delta waves are related with profound sleep, healing, and the subconscious. Gamma waves are related with exceptional performance, wisdom, and transcendence. Hijama cupping therapy increases brain wave synchronization and harmony, as well as mental and physical function. Hijama cupping therapy also raises knowledge and consciousness of oneself, others, and the divine.

The treatment and prevention of spiritual illnesses and disorders

Hijama cupping therapy heals and prevents a wide range of spiritual ailments and conditions, including spiritual emptiness, estrangement, and perplexity.

- Purifying and cleaning the soul and heart. Hijama cupping therapy purifies and cleanses the spirit and heart by removing taiba, which is a term used to describe toxic substances, poisons, waste products, and excess fluids that build up in the body and cause a variety of ailments and problems. The taiba also comprises spiritual impurities such as sins, wicked deeds, poor habits, and negative emotions, which build in the soul and heart and create a variety of spiritual ailments and disorders, including hypocrisy, arrogance, envy, rage, and hatred. Hijama cupping therapy removes taiba from the body and soul while also cleansing the blood and heart.

- Hijama cupping therapy promotes faith and devotion by uniting and aligning the body, mind, and spirit, as well as improving awareness and consciousness of oneself, others, and the divine. Hijama cupping therapy also strengthens faith and devotion by adhering to divine teachings and guidance, such as the Quran, the Sunnah, the Hadith, and the Prophet Muhammad (peace be upon him), who endorsed and performed hijama cupping therapy as a form of prayer and healing. Hijama cupping therapy also strengthens faith and devotion by expressing thanks and praise to the divine, who created and sustains the body, mind, and soul, and bestows the gifts and advantages of Hijama cupping therapy.

The Different Theories and Mechanisms of Hijama Cupping Therapy

Numerous hypotheses and explanations explain the mechanism of Hijama cupping therapy and its effectiveness. The following are a few hypotheses and methods of Hijama cupping therapy:

Endorphin Theory

According to this theory, Hijama cupping therapy causes the production of endorphins, which are natural painkillers and mood enhancers. Endorphins alleviate pain, inflammation, and stress while increasing happiness and relaxation. Endorphins are peptides produced by the pituitary gland and hypothalamus that bind to opioid receptors in the brain and spinal cord, inhibiting the transmission of pain signals. Endorphins also produce feelings of euphoria, enjoyment, and relaxation while lowering tension and anxiety levels. Hijama cupping therapy increases the creation and release of endorphins by generating a suction on the skin with cups and extracting blood and toxins from the tissues beneath. This mechanism activates nerve endings and receptors on the skin and muscles, which convey messages to the brain and spinal cord, resulting in the production of endorphins. This hypothesis describes how Hijama cupping therapy relieves pain and anxiety for a variety of conditions, including acute, chronic, musculoskeletal, and neuropathic pain.

The Gate Control Theory of Pain

According to this theory, Hijama cupping therapy inhibits the passage of pain signals from the nerves to the brain, hence reducing pain, inflammation, and sensitivity while increasing comfort and tolerance. Melzack and Wall presented the gate control theory of pain in 1965, implying that the spinal cord contains a gate or channel that affects pain perception. The gate can be opened or closed by a variety of factors, including the severity, frequency, and kind of pain stimuli, as well as the individual's emotional and cognitive state. When the gate is open, pain impulses can flow from the spinal cord to the brain, resulting in pain perception. When the gate is closed, pain impulses are inhibited or diminished, resulting in decreased or no pain experience. Hijama cupping therapy closes the gate or gateway by activating nerve endings and receptors on the skin and muscles, which send signals to the spinal cord and brain, influencing pain perception. Hijama cupping therapy also effects the person's emotional and cognitive state, lowering stress and anxiety levels while increasing happiness and relaxation, effectively closing the gate or route. This theory explains how Hijama cupping therapy reduces pain intensity and duration by blocking the gate or passage that sends pain signals from peripheral neurons to the central nervous system.

Reflex reaction theory

According to this theory, Hijama cupping therapy stimulates the reflex zones and spots on the skin that are linked to the internal organs and systems, improving organ and system function and balance while treating or preventing a variety of diseases and ailments. The reflex reaction theory is based on the concept of reflexology, which is a type of alternative medicine that uses pressure and massage on reflex zones and points on the feet, hands, and ears that are thought to correspond to internal organs and systems and affect their health and function. Hijama cupping therapy stimulates the skin's reaction zones and points by producing a vacuum with cups and extracting blood and toxins from the underlying tissues. This process activates nerve endings and receptors on the skin and muscles, which send signals to the brain and spinal cord, causing a reflex reaction or response from the body that affects the functions and activities of various organs and systems, including the heart, liver, kidneys, lungs, digestive system, reproductive system, and musculoskeletal system.

This theory explains how hijama cupping therapy affects the blood circulation, immune system, nervous system, endocrine system, and lymphatic system by stimulating the skin's reflex zones and points, as well as how it prevents and treats a variety of diseases and conditions such as diabetes, pain, hypertension, arthritis, asthma, skin problems, infertility, and more.

Prostaglandin Theory

According to this theory, Hijama cupping therapy influences the production and release of prostaglandins, which are hormone-like substances that regulate various physiological processes such as blood pressure, blood clotting, inflammation, and immunity, and thus regulates and normalizes these processes while treating or preventing a variety of diseases and disorders. Prostaglandins are lipid molecules generated from fatty acids that have a variety of physiological functions, including regulation of inflammation, fever, pain, blood clotting, and smooth muscle contraction. Prostaglandins are produced and released by different cells and tissues in the body, including mast cells, platelets, endothelial cells, and smooth muscle cells. Hijama cupping therapy influences prostaglandin formation and release by improving blood flow and oxygen delivery to cells and tissues, as well as eliminating dangerous chemicals, toxins, waste products, and excess fluids from them. Hijama cupping therapy also enhances the creation and release of a variety of anti-inflammatory and analgesic mediators, including endorphins, cortisol, histamine, and serotonin, which influence prostaglandin formation and release. This theory explains how Hijama cupping therapy reduces inflammation and pain by increasing the levels of prostaglandins E2 and F2, which inhibit the synthesis of thromboxane A2 and leukotriene B4, two pro-inflammatory mediators that cause inflammation symptoms such as swelling, redness, heat, and pain.

Taiba Theory

According to this theory, Hijama cupping therapy removes taiba, which is harmful or impure blood and fluids that accumulate in the body as a result of various factors such as diet, lifestyle, environment, or emotions, and cleanses and purifies the body while also treating or preventing various diseases and conditions. The taiba hypothesis is founded on the notion of taiba, which refers to hazardous chemicals, poisons, waste products, and excess fluids that build up in the body and cause a variety of diseases and problems. The taiba also comprises spiritual impurities such as sins, wicked deeds, poor habits, and negative emotions, which build in the soul and heart and create a variety of spiritual ailments and disorders, including hypocrisy, arrogance, envy, rage, and hatred. Hijama cupping therapy removes taiba from both the body and the soul by creating a vacuum on the skin with cups and pulling blood and toxins from the surrounding tissues. This technique eliminates taiba from the blood and tissues while also cleansing and purifying the body and psyche. This theory explains how hijama cupping therapy restores the balance of vital energy or life force by removing the taiba from the body and soul, as well as how it prevents and treats a variety of diseases and conditions, including diabetes, pain, hypertension, arthritis, asthma, skin problems, infertility, and others.

When is hijama applied?

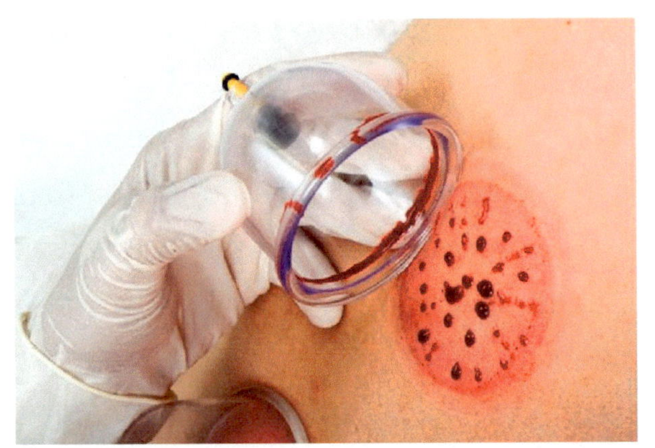

When hijama is required, a treatment plan will be developed; sessions will be held often at first, typically once a month, and then less frequently as needed based on progress. Hijama cleaning may be recommended once every three months for a healthy individual who exercises regularly and eats a balanced diet, especially during the summer and before the change of seasons. We usually wait until the crimson stains from the previous session, known as "Ecchymosis," and the scratches have completely faded before beginning another Hijama therapy session. This typically occurs before two weeks.

Individuals who are unwell or in poor health may need Hijama on a monthly basis before being placed on a quarterly (every three months) regimen. Typically, once every month for three months. When the client's condition is critical, Hijama will be performed biweekly, then monthly, and finally quarterly.

Hijama improves your immune system and protects you from colds and flu during the winter months. Cold temperatures cause our blood vessels to tighten and narrow, boosting blood pressure and the risk of a stroke. Furthermore, the cold can thicken blood, raising the risk of clot formation. Hijama is used in the summer to protect you from the effects of heat on your blood pressure. Both cold and heat cause "flight or fight" reactions, which Hijama aids your body in managing. Hijama, when performed in the spring, can help ease allergy problems by managing Histamine levels. When practiced in the fall, it can help with seasonal depression by allowing your body to release endorphins and serotonin while also preparing your immune system for the oncoming flu and cold season.

Another notion holds that around half of your blood is formed of red blood cells, or erythrocytes. RBCs have an approximate age of 100 days and an average lifespan of 120 days, hence a 90-day hijama interval is recommended. However, aged red blood cells are absorbed by macrophages, filtered by the kidneys, and removed from the body via the spleen and lymph nodes. However, when we are unwell, our systems are unable to fully recycle all of these old and defective red blood cells, causing them to accumulate in specific places of our bodies. These aged red blood cells move throughout our bodies until they reach the capillaries, which occurs when their number increases. Provide oxygen, nutrients, and blood to the cells. They also clear the cells' waste. These capillaries get saturated and clogged, affecting the operation of our organs.

The notion that Hijama is more significant during the summer than during the winter is a prevalent fallacy. In reality, our internal organs maintain a year-round average temperature of approximately 37°. We have an equal demand for Hijama in the winter and summer, particularly for smokers, the elderly, and laborers who are required to spend considerable time seated. Indeed, unanticipated fatalities can result from pulmonary embolism and deep vein thrombosis, both of which are more prevalent during the winter months. This is because we move less and drink less during the winter, which causes our blood vessels' muscle fibers to constrict.

Hijama according to the months of the Hijri Calendar (Islamic or H1: Lunar calendar):

The recommended periods for Hijama are on the 17th, 19th, & 21st days of the month according to the Islamic/ Hijri/ Lunar Calendar.

These Sunnah dates for Hijama have significant significance in Islam religion. The combination of the 17th, 19th, and 21st with Monday, Tuesday, and Thursday are the finest for Hijama.

Cupping therapy is a versatile and effective approach that may be performed at any time, place, or day. It is a natural and effective approach to boost your health, well-being, and performance.

Chapter
06

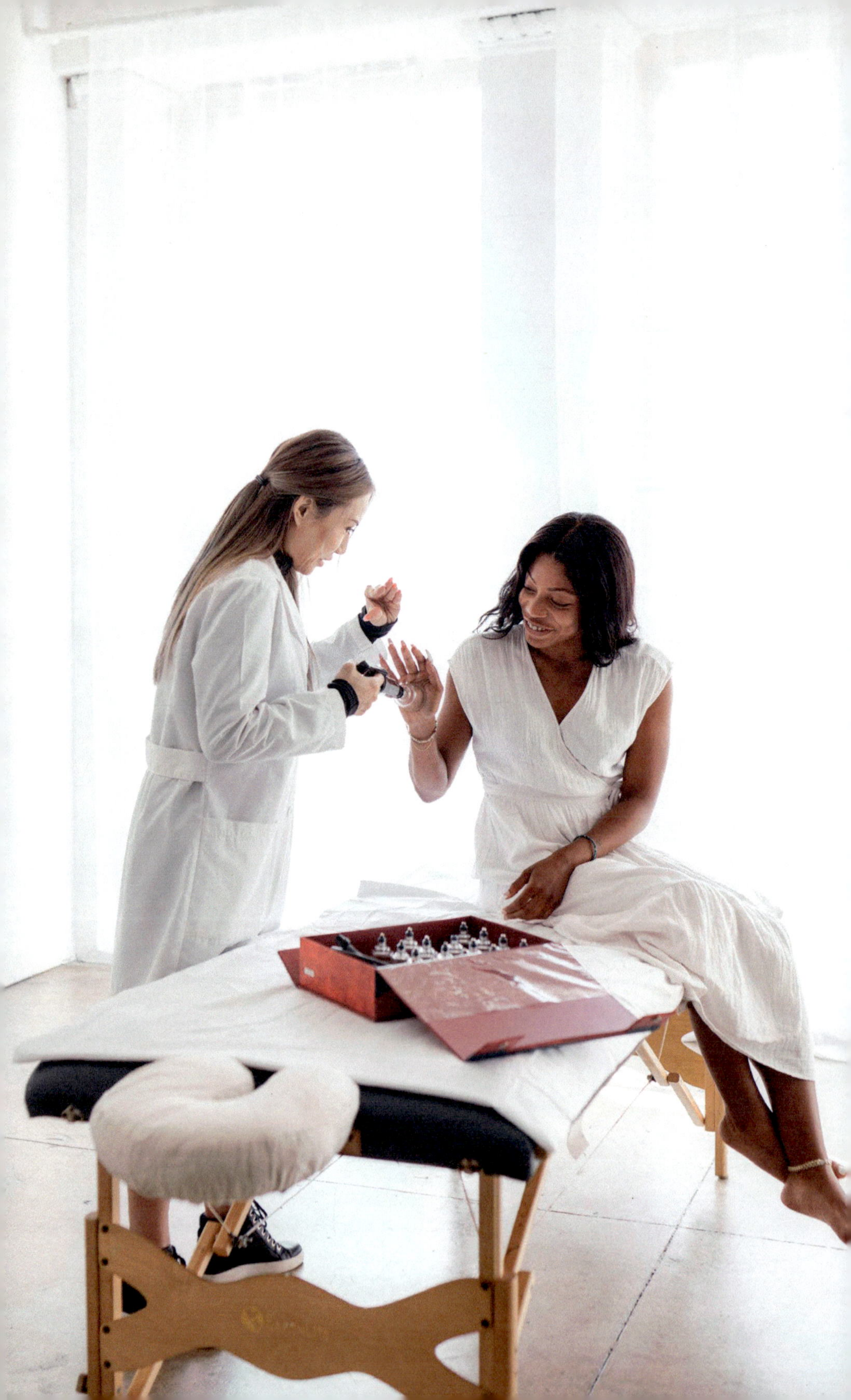

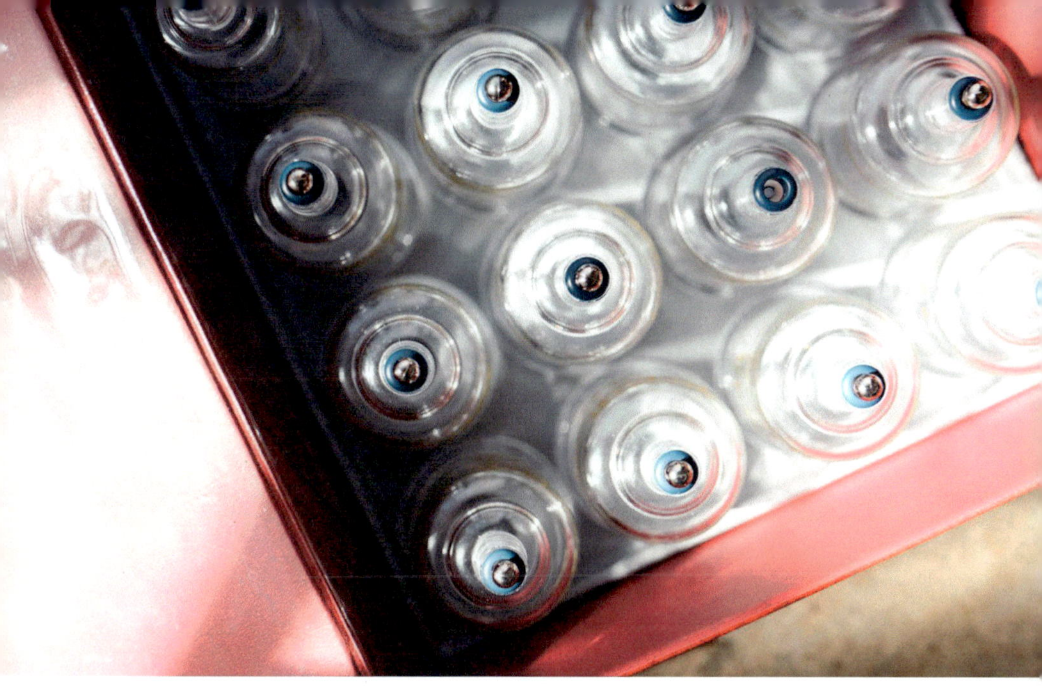

The Science of Cups: A Deep Dive into Hijama Points and Their Benefits

General Hijama Points

General Hijama points are the locations on the body where Hijama can be applied for various health benefits. These points are based on the principles of acupuncture, which is a system of healing that uses needles to stimulate the energy flow in the body. Hijama can activate the same points as acupuncture, but with cups instead of needles. There are many general Hijama points on the body, but some of the most common ones are:

The following are different diseases and ailments, as well as the points at which cupping (Hijama) can be used to cure them. Some of these areas are on nerves while others are on blood arteries. Some are on the power lines (acupuncture), while others are on the back's reflex points. Some are on the lymphatic glands, while others are used to accumulate blood. Some stimulate endocrine secretions, while others boost the immune system. Others aim to strengthen the brain.

Group (A)

Rheumatism (painful joints) (points 1, 55, in addition to all areas of pain).

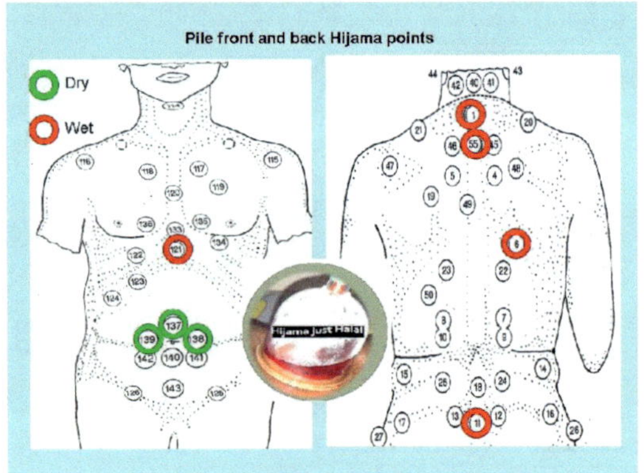

Roughness of knee (points 1, 55, 11, 12, 13 and cupping around the knee and you may add 53, 54).

Oedema (swollen tissue due to build-up of fluid) (points 1, 55, 130, the right and left side of the heel and you may add 9, 10).

Sciatic pain (nerve pain from the buttock which goes down the leg) (for the right leg) (points 1, 55, 11, 12, 26, 51 and places of pain on the leg especially the beginning and the end of the muscle) (for the left leg) (points 1, 55, 11, 13, 27, 52 and places of pain on the leg especially the beginning and the end of the muscle).

Back pain (positions 1, 55 and cupping on both sides of the spine and places of pain).

Neck/shoulder pain (points 1, 55, 40, 20, 21 and places of pain).

Gout (swollen joints due to excess uric acid) (points 1, 55, 28, 29, 30, 31, 121 and places of pain).

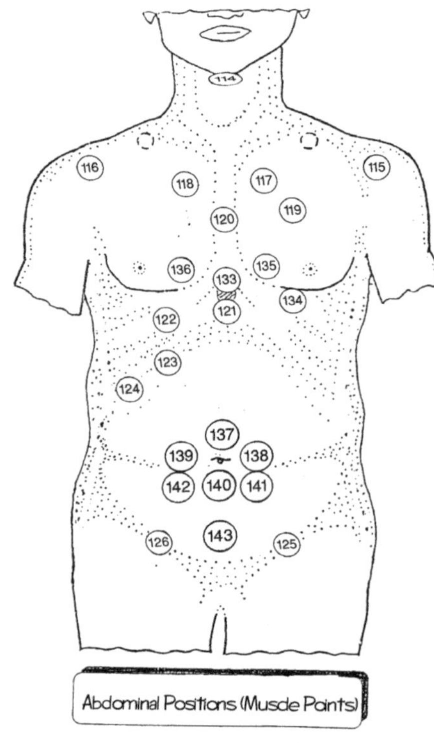

Rheumatoid Arthritis (points 1, 55, 120, 49, 36 and all large and small joints).

Paralysis of one half of the body (Hemiplegia) (points 1, 55, 11, 12, 13, 34 or 35 and all the injured joints, massage daily).

Paralysis of all four limbs (Quadriplegia) (points 1, 55, 11, 12, 13, 34, 35, 36 and all body joints and daily massage).

Immune system deficiency (points 1, 55, 120, and 49).

Muscle spasm several dry cupping around the affected muscle.

Poor blood circulation (points 1, 55, 11 and ten cups on both sides of the spine from the top to the bottom in addition to taking a teaspoon of pure organic, raw, apple cider vinegar and honey every other day).

Tingling arms (points 1, 55, 40, 20, 21, arm muscles and affected joints).

Tingling feet (points 1, 55, 11, 12, 13, 26, 27, feet joints and affected muscles).

Abdominal pain (points 1, 55, 7, 8 and dry cupping on 137, 138, 139, 140, as well as dry cupping on the back opposite to the pain). (Dry Cupping means without any incisions/ scratches).

Group (B)

Important Note: The following points are arranged according to their importance. Sometimes, the cupping therapist does not need to use all of the points and sometimes he/she has to use them all, depending on the condition of the disease.

Hemorrhoids (swollen vessels around anus) (points 1, 55, 121, 11, 6 and dry cupping on 137, 138, 139).

Anal Fistula (opening in skin near anus, due to formation of a channel through which fluid leaks) (points 1, 55, 6, 11, 12, 13 and cupping around the anus and above the fistula hole).

Prostate and Erectile dysfunction, ED (male impotence and urinary difficulty due to enlarged prostate gland) (points 1, 55, 6, 11, 12, 13) and you may add for ED 125, 126, 131 on both legs, and dry cupping on 140, 143.

Chronic coughs and lung diseases (points 1, 55, 4, 5, 120, 49, 115, 116, 9, 10, 117, 118, 135, 136, and two cups below both knees).

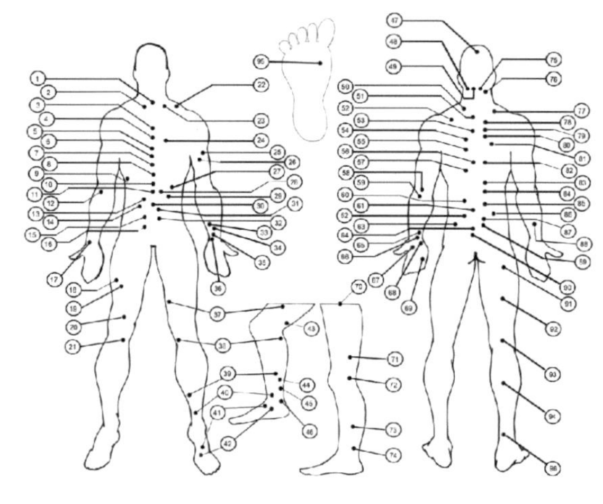

Hypertension (high blood pressure) (points 1, 55, 2, 3, 11, 12, 13, 101, 32, 6, 48, 9, 10, 7, 8, and you may replace 2, 3 with 43, 44).

Stomach problems and ulcers (points 1, 55, 7, 8, 50, 41, 42 and dry cupping on 137, 138, 139, and 140).

Renal (kidney) disease (points 1, 55, 9, 10, 41, 42 and dry cupping on 137,140).

Irritable bowel syndrome (abdominal cramps and discomfort characterized by bloating and trapped wind and alternating bouts of diarrhea and constipation, often related to anxiety) (points 1, 55, 6, 48, 7, 8, 14, 15, 16, 17, 18, 45, 46 and dry cupping on 137).

Chronic constipation (long term difficulty with opening bowels) (points 1, 55, 11, 12, 13, 28, 29, 30, and 31).

Diarrhea (dry cupping on 137, 138, 139, and 140).

Involuntary urination (bed wetting) (after the age of five: dry cupping on 137, 138, 139, 140, 142, 143, 125, and 126).

Depression, withdrawal, insomnia (inability to sleep), psychological conditions and nervousness (points 1, 55, 6, 11, 32 and below the knees).

Angiospasm and Arteriosclerosis (narrowing of the blood vessels due to muscular spasm or fatty deposits) (points 1, 55, 11) (cupping points are on the places of pain in addition to a teaspoon of pure, organic, raw, apple cider vinegar and honey every other day).

Inflammation in the lining of the stomach (gastritis) (points 1, 55, and 121).

Excessive sleep (points 1, 55, and 36) in addition to a teaspoon of pure, organic, raw, apple cider vinegar and honey every other day).

Food allergies (one dry cup using a light suction directly on the umbilicus pit [belly button]).

Sores, leg and thigh abscesses (pus filled spots) and itching of iliac fossae (itching in hip area) (points 1, 55, 129, 120).

Group (C)

Important Note: The following points are arranged according to their importance. Sometimes, the cupping therapist does not need to use all of the points and sometimes he/she has to use them all depending on the condition of the disease.

Heart disease (points 1, 55, 19, 119, 7, 8, 46, 46, 47, 133, and 134).

Diabetes (points 1, 55, 6, 7, 8, 22, 23, 24, 25, 120, 49) note: the area

of cupping should be applied with black seed oil or honey for 3 days.

Liver and gall bladder disease (points 1, 55, 6, 48, 41, 42, 46, 51, 122, 123, 124 and 5 cups on the right, outer leg).

Varicose veins (enlarged, unsightly superficial veins) on the legs (points 1, 55, 28, 29, 30, 31, 132 and around the veins but NOT over the veins).

Varicocele (enlarged unsightly veins on scrotum of male) (points 1, 55, 6, 11, 12, 13, 28, 29, 30, 31, 125, 126).

Elephantiasis (swollen leg due to blockage of lymph channels) note: the patient should rest for 2 days before cupping. He/She should also raise his/her affected leg up and then place it in warm water for two hours prior to cupping (points 1, 55, 11, 12, 13, 120, 49, 121 and around the affected leg from the top of the leg to the bottom in addition to 125, 126, 53, 54).

Skin diseases (points 1, 55, 49, 120, 129, 6, 7, 8, 11 and cupping on the affected areas).

Overweight (points 1, 55, 9, 10, 120, 49 and areas of desired weight loss), daily massage cupping over area of desired weight loss.

Underweight (points 1, 55, and 121).

Cellulite daily massage cupping over affected area.

Infertility (points 1, 55, 6, 11, 12, 13, 120, 49, 125, 126, 143, 41, and 42).

Thyroid disease (points 1, 55, 41, and 42).

Group (D)

Headaches (points 1, 55, 2, 3) and you may replace points 2, 3 with 43, 44. If it is caused by eye strain add 104, 105 and 36. If it is caused by nasal sinuses add 102, 103 and 114. If it is caused by high blood pressure add 11, 101 and 32. If it is caused by constipation add 28, 29, 30 and 31. If it is caused by a cold add 120, 4 and 5. If it is caused by a stomach ache add 7, 8. If it is caused by the kidneys add 9, 10. If it is caused by menstruation for women add 11, 12 and 13. If it is caused by gall bladder and liver add 6, 48. If it is caused by the spine column perform cupping on the spine. If it is caused by tension add 6, 11 and 32. If it is caused by anemia add 120, 49 and take one teaspoon of black honey (molasses) with a quarter of a teaspoon of ground fenugreek and 7 ground black seeds daily. If the headache is due to tumors in

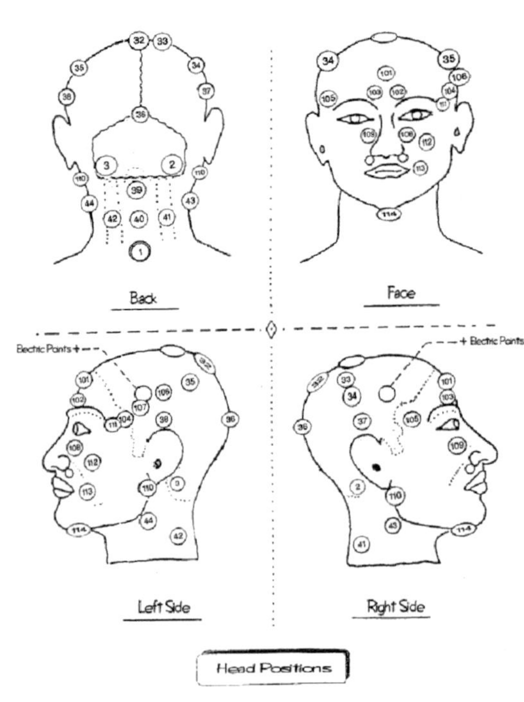

the brain, cupping should be performed on the area of pain on the head).

Migraine (severe headache associated with nausea and visual disturbance) (points 1, 55, 2, 3, 106 and area of pain).

Diseases of the eyes (retina, eye disorder, blurred vision, atrophy of the eye nerves, glaucoma (Blue Water), cataract (White Water) and weak eye, eye inflammation and secretion of tears and eye sensitivity (points 1, 55, 36, 101, 104, 105, 9, 10, 34, 35, above the eyebrows and on the hair line above the forehead).

Tonsils, throat, gums, teeth, and the middle ear problems (dizziness, nausea and ringing in ears) (points 1, 55, 20, 21, 41, 42, 120, 49, 114, 43, 44).

Weakness of hearing and inflammation of hearing nerve, tinnitus (ringing sensation in ears) (points 1, 55, 20, 21, 37, 38 and behind the ear).

Nasal sinuses (points 1, 55, 102, 103, 108, 109, 36, 14 and on the hair line).

Neuritis (inflammation) of the fifth and seventh nerves (points 1, 55, 110, 111, 112, 113, 114 and on the affected area).

To stimulate the system of perception (encourage awareness) (points 1, 55, 2, 3, 32).

Clinical Memory Loss (important: if point 39 is cupped unnecessarily it may cause damage to the memory. Also its unnecessary repetition may increase memory loss (point 39 occipital prominence).

Mute (unable to speak) (points 1, 55, 36, 33, 107, and 114).

To help stop smoking (points 1, 55, 106, 11, and 32).

Convulsion (fits) (points 1, 55, 101, 36, 32, 107 on sides, 114, 11, 12, 13).

For the treatment of mental retardation (points 1, 55, (101 only once) 36, 32, 2, 3, 120, 49, 11, 12, 13).

Atrophy (loss) of brain cells (oxygen deficiency) (points 1, 55, 101, 36, 32, 34, 35, and 11 and perform cupping on the joints, muscles and neck, 43 and 44 on the front and back. Eat honey and royal jelly. Perform massage cupping daily).

Group (E) Gynecological

Important warning: pregnant women should avoid cupping during pregnancy except if they are over-due and wish to go into labor. In this case, they should have dry and massage cupping between the knee and ankle on both legs. Cupping a pregnant woman may cause miscarriage.

Hemorrhage (vaginal bleeding) (points 1, 55, (3 dry cups under each breast daily until bleeding ceases).

Amenorrhea (absence of periods) (points 1, 55, 129, (131 from the outside), 135, 136).

Brownish Secretion 3 dry cups under each breast daily until secretion ceases (points 1, 55, 120, 49, 11, 12, 13 and 143). If secretion has no smell, no color or itching, perform cupping on (points 1, 55, 9, 10, 41, 42, 11, 12, 13, 143).

Menstruation (period) problems (points 1, 55 (dry cupping on 125, 126, 137, 138, 139, 140, 141, 142, 143).

To stimulate the ovaries (points 1, 55, 11, (dry cupping on 125, 126).

Pain after a uterus (womb) operation, menstrual (period) pain, the problems of ligation of the fallopian tube (tube being tied/blocked), milk existence in the breast without being pregnant and menopausal symptoms (depression, nervousness, psychological conditions, acute uterus) (points 1, 55, 6, 48, 11, 12, 13, 120, 49) (Dry Cupping on 125, 126). To regulate the menses, it is preferred to perform cupping on the second day of the menses.

Cupping places on the back

1, the shoulder, the seventh vertebra (bone of spine) of the neck.

2 & 3, the area between the ears, the back of the head where hair grows or on the sides of the neck.

4 & 5, the air door between the two ribs upwards in the branching of the tracheae (main windpipe) and the bronchus (smaller windpipe).

6, the gall bladder at the peripheral of the right rib toward the spine.

7 & 8, on the stomach place at the middle of the back opposite to the stomach on the spinal sides.

9 & 10, the kidney center under 7 & 8 on the middle of the back.

11, lumbar vertebrae – a prominent bone at the lower back of the vertebra column.

12 & 13, on the sides of 11, slightly upward, 5cm away from the spine.

14, 15, 16 & 17, the colon, almost on the colon corners from the back and 18ofthe middle of the spine.

19, the heart, opposite to the heart from the back and almost on the left rib side.

20 & 21, tonsils triangle that lies in the area between the neck and the shoulder with a slight bending to the back.

22 & 23, above the pancreas gland under the rib end.

24 & 25, at the beginning of the lower half of the back.

26 & 27, bilaterally at the sides of the iliac bone.

28, 29, 30 & 31, at the upper part of the buttocks.

32, on the middle of the head.

33, on the right part of the hair near the forehead or the hair line.

34 & 35, the right and left part of the brain (at the temporal sides of the brain) as well as the occipital bone.

36, the cerebellum (occipital) prominent bone on the head.

37 & 38, nearly 3cm above the ears.

39, prominent occipital bone, the deep area at the back of the head where cupping is prohibited, except in necessary cases.

40, in the middle of the back of the neck.

41 & 42, on the back of the head to the right and the left.

43 & 44, the sides of the neck.

45 & 46, nearly 3cm above the air trachea (4-5).

47, on the left shoulder in addition to the heart.

48, on the right rib from upward, complementary to the gall bladder knot.

49, the immunity area from the back, between the two scapulae (shoulder blades).

50, 6cm slightly above 8, for stomach ulcers.

51 & 52, the two thigh bones (femur), from both sides.

53 & 54, the inner part of the knee from the back.

55, almost 3cm under the shoulder.

Cupping places on the face and abdomen

101, the forehead on the place of worship in praying and it is better not to repeat it.

102 & 103, above the eyebrows from the inner part of the nasal sinuses.

104 & 105, on both sides of the brows and slightly upward for headaches and sight.

106, almost 6cm above the left ear to help give up smoking.

107, nearly 4cm above the cheeks to assist in speech.

108 & 109, on the sides of the nose for nasal sinuses.

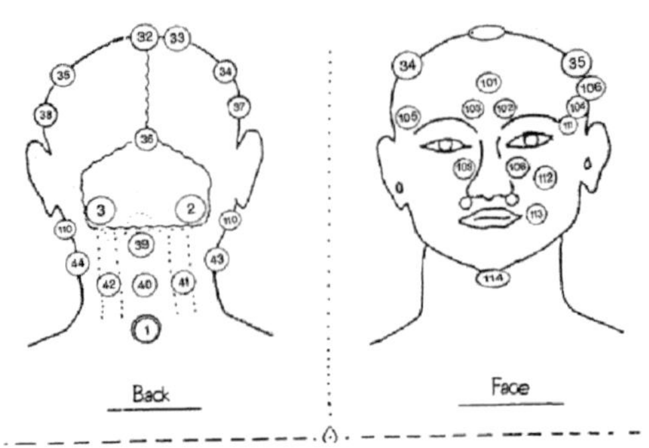

110, under the ear from the right and left.

111, 112 & 113, near the eye and the cheek and near the

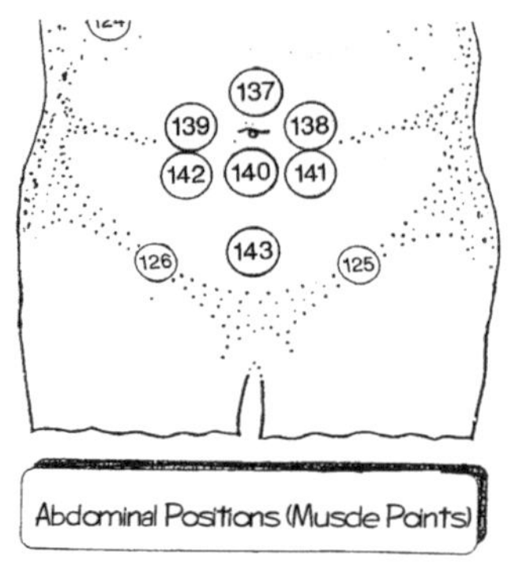

lip to treat the fifth and sixth nerve.

114, under the chin and it has many benefits.

115 & 116, under the ends of the clavicle (collar bone) from the outside and on the shoulders.

117 & 118, under the clavicle (collar bone) from the inside, on the chest.

119, the heart, under the middle of the left clavicle (collar bone) using four fingers of the patient himself.

120, sternum bone (breastplate), in the middle of the chest.

121, first part of the stomach directly under the chest bone.

122, 123 & 124, above the liver, right of the belly.

125 & 126, between the belly and the thigh near the pubic hair area for involuntary urination, infertility...etc.

127 & 128, on the inner part of the thighs.

129, on the back of the feet to the right.

130, on the sides of the heel from inside and outside for edema.

131, above the heel bone nearly 5cm from the outside.

132, varicocele.

133, almost 2cm above the stomach mouth and near the end of the chest bone.

134, under the left breast.

135 & 136, 5cm away from the breast nipple from the inside for the lungs.

137, 138, 139 & 140, above, right, left and under the umbilicus (belly button).

141, & 142, Right and left of 140.

143, above the bladder.

Indications of Hijama and points according to indications

Hijama for enuresis:

Hijama for enuresis is a type of Hijama that focuses on the urinary system, including the bladder, kidneys, and lower abdomen. Enuresis is the involuntary loss of pee, which occurs primarily at night in children and adults. It can be caused by a variety of factors, including psychological stress, hormonal imbalance, urinary tract infection, or neurological disorders. Hijama for enuresis can have various benefits, including:

Improving bladder and kidney function

Hijama for enuresis can help with bladder and kidney function by increasing blood flow and lymphatic drainage to these organs. It can also control urine output and fluid balance in the body. This advantage is provided via points on the forehead, chest, stomach, and lower back.

Relieving urinary tract infection and irritation

Hijama for enuresis can help with urinary tract infection and inflammation by removing germs and toxins from the urinary system. It can help alleviate the discomfort and burning sensations associated with the illness. The sites for this benefit include the lower back, lower abdomen, and inner ankle.

Calming the nerves and emotions

Hijama for enuresis helps soothe nerves and emotions by activating the parasympathetic nervous system and endorphins. It can also help to regulate mood and hormones, as well as ease anxiety and despair. The spots for this benefit are the top of the head point, the forehead point, the heart point, and the inner wrist points.

Hijama points for menstrual irregularities and unpleasant menstruation:

Hijama points for menstrual irregularity and painful menstruation are those associated with the female reproductive system, such as the ovaries, uterus, and lower abdomen. Menstrual irregularity refers to abnormal variations in the length, frequency, or flow of the menstrual cycle. Painful menstruation is the cramping or painful discomfort in the lower abdomen or back during or before the menstrual cycle. Hormonal imbalance, ovarian cysts, endometriosis, or fibroids are some of the possible causes of these diseases. Hijama points for menstrual irregularity and uncomfortable menstruation can have various advantages, including:

Balancing hormones and menstrual cycles

Hijama points for menstrual irregularity and painful menstruation might help balance hormones and regulate the menstrual cycle by stimulating the ovaries and pituitary gland. It can also control ovulation and menstruation and help prevent or cure illnesses like polycystic ovarian syndrome, amenorrhea, and dysmenorrhea. This advantage is provided by the points situated on the lower belly, lower back, inner ankle, inner knee, and top of foot.

Strengthening the uterus and blood

Hijama points for menstrual irregularities and uncomfortable menstruation can strengthen the uterus and blood by feeding the endometrium and blood vessels. It can also help prevent or treat diseases including anemia, severe bleeding, and clotting. This advantage is available in the following points: lower belly, navel, inner knee, upper back, and liver.

Harmonizing qi and blood

Hijama points for menstrual irregularities and uncomfortable menstruation can help to balance the qi and blood by clearing stagnation and blockages in the pelvic area. It can also help the reproductive system repair and function properly. The points for this benefit include the navel, stomach, lower thigh, chest, and outer knee.

Hijama points for asthma:

Hijama points for asthma are the points related to the respiratory system, such as the lungs, the chest, and the back. Asthma is a chronic inflammatory condition of the airways that causes wheezing, coughing, shortness of breath, and chest tightness. It can be triggered by various factors, such as allergens, pollution, exercise, or stress. Hijama points for asthma can have several benefits, such as:

- **Expanding the chest and the lungs**

Hijama points for asthma can expand the chest and the lungs by creating a negative pressure inside the cups. This can increase the oxygen intake and the blood circulation to the respiratory system. The points for this benefit are the chest point, the throat point, the upper lung points, the lower lung points, and the upper back points.

- **Relieving the cough and the asthma**

Hijama points for asthma can relieve the cough and the asthma by clearing the phlegm and the congestion from the respiratory tract and the lungs. It can also reduce the inflammation and the irritation of the airways and the bronchi. The points for this benefit are the navel point, the lower leg points, the elbow crease points, the wrist crease points, and the upper back points.

- **Calming the emotions and the nerves**

Hijama points for asthma can calm the emotions and the nerves by activating the vagus nerve and the parasympathetic nervous system. It can also balance the mood and the hormones and relieve anxiety and depression. The points for this benefit are the top of the head point, the forehead point, the heart point, and the inner wrist points.

Hijama Cupping Therapy for depression and psychological sicknesses, acne and pimples:

Hijama for depression and psychological illnesses, as well as acne and pimples, is a sort of Hijama that is conducted on points connected to the nervous system, endocrine system, and skin, including the head, neck, and back. Depression and psychological illnesses are mental impairments that cause a variety of behavioral changes and lower one's quality of life. Acne and pimples are inflammatory skin conditions characterized by redness, swelling, and pus-filled lumps. These diseases can have a variety of origins, including genetic, environmental, hormonal, and emotional aspects. Hijama for depression and psychiatric illnesses, acne and pimples can provide a number of benefits, including

Improving mental clarity and concentration

Hijama for depression, psychiatric illnesses, acne, and pimples might increase mental clarity and attention by increasing blood flow and oxygen to the brain. It can also purge the mind of bad thoughts and emotions, boosting awareness and intuition. The points for this benefit are at the top of the head, the forehead, between the brows, and on the nose bridge.

Relieving depression and psychological illnesses

Hijama for depression and psychological disorders, acne, and pimples can alleviate depression and psychological problems by releasing tension and spasms in the muscles and nerves of the head and neck. It can also regulate hormones and neurotransmitters that influence pain perception and mood. This advantage is available through the following points: back of the head, shoulder, side of the neck, and front of the neck.

Purifying the skin and blood

Hijama for depression, psychological illnesses, acne, and pimples can cleanse the skin and blood by removing toxins and waste from the body and mind. It can also improve your complexion and vision, as well as treat skin conditions including acne, eczema, and psoriasis. The spots for this benefit are the upper back points, the liver point, the kidney point, and the lower back points.

Hijama Cupping Therapy for ankylosing spondylitis:

Hijama for ankylosing spondylitis is a type of Hijama that focuses on the musculoskeletal system, including the spine, hips, and sacroiliac joints. Ankylosing spondylitis is a chronic inflammatory illness that primarily affects the spine but may also affect other joints. It causes discomfort, stiffness, and restricted movement in the spine and can develop to vertebral fusion. It can have a variety of reasons, including genetic, environmental, and immunological factors. Hijama for ankylosing spondylitis can have various benefits, including:

Relaxing the muscles and the tendons

Hijama for ankylosing spondylitis helps relax muscles and tendons by creating negative pressure within the cups. This can help to increase joint and limb flexibility. The points for this benefit include the tailbone, lower back, mid back, upper back, and neck.

Relieving pain and inflammation

Hijama for ankylosing spondylitis can help with pain and inflammation by relieving pressure and swelling in the spine and joints. It can also regulate the hormones and neurotransmitters that influence pain perception and inflammation. This benefit is available at the kidney, lower back, sacroiliac joint, hip, and lower back spots.

Stimulating Healing and Recovery

Hijama for ankylosing spondylitis can promote healing and recovery by boosting the immune system and defense against infections and diseases. It can also help in the regeneration and repair of damaged tissues and bones.

Hijama Cupping Therapy for Herniated disc - Lumbar Pains Skin illnesses:

Hijama for herniated discs, lumbar aches, and skin problems is a type of Hijama done on locations connected to the spine, lower back, and skin, such as the tailbone, lower back, and upper back. A herniated disc occurs when the soft inner component of the disc between the vertebrae bulges out and presses on the nerves, resulting in discomfort, numbness, or weakness in the back or legs. Skin ailments include acne, eczema, psoriasis, and infections. Hijama for herniated discs, lumbar aches, and skin problems can have various benefits, including:

Relieving pain and inflammation

Hijama for herniated discs, lumbar aches, and skin disorders can help reduce pain and inflammation by lowering pressure and swelling in the spine and nerves. It can also regulate the hormones and neurotransmitters that influence pain perception and inflammation. This advantage is available at the tailbone, lower back, sacroiliac joint, hip, and lower back locations.

Improving spinal alignment and posture

Hijama for herniated discs, lumbar discomfort, and skin illnesses can help with spinal alignment and posture by relaxing the muscles and tendons that support the spine. It can also help to prevent or treat diseases like scoliosis, kyphosis, and lordosis, which impact the curvature of the spine. This advantage is available in the lower back, middle back, upper back, and neck locations.

Purifying skin and blood, as well as using a Hijama to alleviate lumbar pain from herniated discs. Skin illnesses can cleanse the skin and blood by eliminating toxins and waste from the body and psyche. It can also enhance complexion and vision, as well as treat skin conditions like acne, eczema, psoriasis, and infections. The spots for this benefit are the upper back points, the liver point, the kidney point, and the lower back points.

Hijama Cupping Therapy for Vascular stenosis, vein toughness Epilepsy Fibromyalgia:

Hijama for vascular stenosis or vein stiffness Epilepsy fibromyalgia is a sort of Hijama that targets places connected to the circulatory, neurological, and muscular systems, such as the chest, neck, and legs. Vascular stenosis is a narrowing of the blood vessels that restricts blood flow to the organs and tissues. Vein stiffness is the lack of elasticity in the veins, which affects blood pressure and cardiac function. Epilepsy is a neurological illness that produces recurring seizures as a result of aberrant electrical activity in the brain. Fibromyalgia is a chronic disorder that causes widespread pain, exhaustion, and cognitive impairment. Hijama for vascular stenosis, vein stiffness, epilepsy, or fibromyalgia can have various benefits, including:

Improving blood circulation and oxygenation

Hijama for vascular stenosis, vein stiffness, epilepsy, and fibromyalgia improves blood circulation and oxygenation by creating negative pressure inside the cups. This may boost oxygen intake and blood flow to the organs and tissues. This advantage is provided by spots on the chest, neck, upper and lower lungs, and upper back.

Relieving convulsions and agony.

Hijama for vascular stenosis, vein stiffness, epilepsy, and fibromyalgia can help decrease seizures and pain by removing phlegm and congestion from the neurological system and muscles. It can also minimize inflammation and irritation to the nerves and fibers. The points for this benefit are the navel, lower thigh, elbow, wrist, and upper back.

Calming emotions and nerves

Hijama for vascular stenosis or vein stiffness Fibromyalgia can relax the emotions and nerves by activating the vagus nerve and the parasympathetic nervous system. It can also help to regulate mood and hormones, as well as ease anxiety and despair. This benefit can be obtained by spots on the top of the head, forehead, heart, and inner wrists.

Hijama Cupping Therapy for Restless foot syndrome Multiple sclerosis (MS):

Hijama for restless foot syndrome multiple sclerosis (MS) is a type of Hijama that focuses on the feet, legs, and immune system, including the inner ankle, lower thigh, and upper back. Restless foot syndrome is characterized by uncomfortable feelings in the feet, such as tingling, crawling, or itching, as well as an impulse to move them. Multiple sclerosis (MS) is a chronic autoimmune illness that destroys the nerves' protective layer, causing issues with vision, mobility, feeling, and cognition. Hijama for restless foot syndrome multiple sclerosis (MS) can have various benefits, including:

Relaxing the feet and legs

Hijama for restless foot syndrome multiple sclerosis (MS) can help to relax the feet and legs by creating negative pressure inside the cups. This can help to increase joint and limb flexibility. The points for this benefit include the inner ankle, lower leg, knee, and hip.

Relieving symptoms and the course of MS

Hijama for restless foot syndrome multiple sclerosis (MS) can alleviate symptoms and slow the progression of the disease by lowering pressure and swelling in the nerves and brain. It can also regulate the hormones and neurotransmitters that influence nerve function and inflammation. This benefit is available at the kidney, lower back, sacroiliac joint, hip, and lower back spots.

Stimulating Healing and Recovery

Hijama for restless foot syndrome multiple sclerosis (MS) can help with healing and recovery by boosting the immune system and defending against viruses and diseases. It can also help regenerate and mend damaged nerves and tissues. The advantage can be gained by spots on the upper back, liver, spleen, and lower back.

Hijama Cupping Therapy for Chronic Fatigue (Tiredness):

Hijama for chronic fatigue (tiredness) is a type of Hijama that is applied to locations connected to energy, metabolism, and sleep, such as the forehead, stomach, and lower back. Chronic fatigue (tiredness) is a syndrome characterized by persistent and unexplained exhaustion that impairs daily activities and quality of life. Stress, depression, illness, and hormone imbalance are some of the possible causes. Hijama for chronic fatigue (tiredness) can have various benefits, including:

Boosting energy and vitality

Hijama for chronic fatigue (tiredness) can improve energy and vitality by increasing blood flow and oxygen to the brain and body. It can also purge the mind of bad thoughts and emotions, boosting awareness and intuition. The points for this benefit are at the top of the head, the forehead, between the brows, and on the nose bridge.

Improving metabolism and digestion

Hijama for chronic fatigue (tiredness) can help with metabolism and digestion by stimulating the stomach and spleen. It can also manage appetite and weight and help to prevent or treat illnesses like obesity, diabetes, and thyroid disorders. The points for this benefit are the lower abdomen, navel, stomach, and spleen.

Enhancing sleep and relaxation

Hijama for chronic fatigue (tiredness) can help you sleep and relax by activating the pineal gland and melatonin. It can also help to regulate the circadian rhythm and sleep cycle, as well as cure insomnia and other sleep disorders. This advantage is provided by the locations on the top of the head, forehead, heart, and inner wrists.

Hijama Cupping Therapy for Migraine Tinnitus:

Hijama for migraine tinnitus is a sort of Hijama that focuses on the head, ears, and neurological system, including the back of the head, the side of the neck, and the upper back. Migraine is a severe, recurring headache that is frequently accompanied by nausea, vomiting, and sensitivity to light and sound. Tinnitus is a ringing or buzzing sound in the ears that can be either continuous or intermittent. Stress, trauma, infection, or a neurological problem are all potential causes of both conditions. Hijama for migraine tinnitus can have various benefits, including:

Balancing hormones and neurotransmitters.

Hijama for migraine tinnitus can help to regulate hormones and neurotransmitters that influence pain perception and mood management. It can also reduce tension, worry, and sadness, all of which can exacerbate migraine and tinnitus symptoms. This advantage is available through the following points: back of the head, shoulder, side of the neck, and front of the neck.

Stimulating Healing and Recovery

Hijama for migraine tinnitus can help with healing and rehabilitation by boosting the immune system and defending against infections and diseases. It can also help with the regeneration and repair of damaged nerves and tissues in the head and ears. This benefit can be found at the upper back, liver, kidney, and lower back areas.

Hijama Cupping Therapy for Adolescent Leadership and the Relationship between the Right and Left Brain:

Hijama for adolescent leadership and right-left brain relationship is a sort of Hijama that is done on places associated with the brain, nervous system, and personality, such as the top of the head, forehead, and back of the head. Leadership is the ability to influence, encourage, and inspire others to work toward a common objective. Adolescence is a pivotal phase in development, during which the brain undergoes considerable changes that affect cognitive, emotional, and social functioning. The right and left hemispheres of the brain play distinct functions and talents, and their integration and balance are critical for peak performance and well-being.

Hijama for leadership in adolescence and the right-left brain link can have various benefits, including:

Enhancing cognitive and creative abilities

Hijama for leadership in adolescence and the right-left brain link can improve cognitive and creative abilities by increasing blood flow and oxygen to the brain and body. It can also purge the mind of bad thoughts and emotions, boosting awareness and intuition. The points for this benefit are at the top of the head, the forehead, between the brows, and on the nose bridge.

Balancing personality and emotions

Hijama for adolescent leadership and the right-left brain interaction can help balance personality and emotions by activating the pineal gland and melatonin. It can also regulate mood and hormones, reducing stress, anxiety, and sadness. This advantage is available through the following points: back of the head, shoulder, side of the neck, and front of the neck.

Developing leadership and communication skills

Hijama for leadership in adolescence, along with the right-left brain link, can help to build leadership and communication abilities by increasing confidence and charisma. It can also improve verbal and nonverbal communication skills, as well as interpersonal interactions. This benefit is available in the throat, chest, heart, and inner wrist points.

Hijama Cupping therapy for Infertility or oligospermia:

Hijama for infertility or oligospermia is a type of Hijama that is applied to spots connected to the reproductive system, hormonal system, and fertility, such as the lower belly, lower back, and inner ankle. Infertility is defined as the failure to conceive a child after one year of regular unprotected intercourse. Oligospermia is a disorder characterized by decreased sperm count or quality, which impacts male fertility. Hijama for infertility or oligospermia can have various benefits, including:

Improving sperm production and motility

Hijama for infertility or oligospermia can increase sperm production and motility by stimulating the testicles and epididymis. It can help manage testosterone and estrogen levels, as well as prevent or treat sperm-quality-affecting illnesses including as obesity, diabetes, and thyroid disorders. The points for this benefit are the lower abdomen, navel, stomach, and spleen.

Enhancing blood circulation and oxygenation

Hijama for infertility or oligospermia can improve blood circulation and oxygenation by creating negative pressure within the cups. This may boost oxygen intake and blood flow to the organs and tissues. This advantage is provided by spots on the chest, neck, upper and lower lungs, and upper back.

Stimulating Healing and Recovery

Hijama for infertility or oligospermia can help with healing and rehabilitation by boosting the immune system and defending against infections and diseases. It can also help in the regeneration and repair of damaged tissues and organs. This benefit can be found at the upper back, liver, kidney, and lower back places.

Hijama Cupping therapy for High Blood Pressure:

Hijama for high blood pressure is a type of Hijama that is applied to locations associated with the heart, blood vessels, and blood pressure, such as the chest, upper back, and lower back. High blood pressure, often known as hypertension, is a disorder in which the blood's force on the arterial walls is excessive, causing damage to the heart, brain, kidneys, and other organs. Hijama for high blood pressure has various benefits, including:

Lowering blood pressure and cholesterol levels

Hijama for high blood pressure can reduce blood volume and viscosity, lowering blood pressure and cholesterol levels. It can also balance the hormones and neurotransmitters that control blood pressure and inflammation. This advantage applies to the chest, upper back, liver, and lower back locations.

Relaxing the blood vessels and muscles

Hijama for high blood pressure can relax the blood vessels and muscles by creating negative pressure within the cups. This can help to increase joint and limb flexibility. The points for this benefit include the inner ankle, lower leg, knee, and hip.

Calming emotions and nerves

Hijama for high blood pressure can soothe the emotions and nerves by activating the vagus nerve and the parasympathetic nervous system. It can also regulate mood and hormones, reducing stress, anxiety, and sadness. This advantage is provided by the locations on the top of the head, forehead, heart, and inner wrists.

Hijama Cupping therapy for Forgetfulness or Dysmnesia:

Hijama for forgetfulness or dysmnesia is a type of Hijama that is applied to places associated with memory, cognition, and learning, such as the top of the head, the forehead, and the rear of the head. Forgetfulness, also known as dysmnesia, is a condition that impairs or eliminates the ability to recall or retain information. Stress, trauma, infection, and neurological disorders are some of the possible causes. Hijama for forgetfulness or dysmnesia can have various benefits, including:

Improving memory and recall

Hijama for forgetfulness or dysmnesia can help with memory and recall by increasing blood flow and oxygen to the brain and body. It can also purge the mind of bad thoughts and emotions, boosting awareness and intuition. The points for this benefit are at the top of the head, the forehead, between the brows, and on the nose bridge.

Enhancing cognitive and creative abilities

Hijama for forgetfulness or dysmnesia can improve cognitive and creative abilities by stimulating the right and left hemispheres of the brain and promoting their integration and balance. It can also improve verbal and nonverbal communication skills, as well as interpersonal interactions. This advantage is available through the following points: back of the head, shoulder, side of the neck, and front of the neck.

Developing learning and focus skills

Hijama for forgetfulness or dysmnesia can improve learning and focus by activating the pineal gland and melatonin. It can also help to regulate the circadian rhythm and sleep cycle, as well as cure insomnia and other sleep disorders. This advantage is provided by the locations on the top of the head, forehead, heart, and inner wrists.

Hijama Cupping therapy for the prostate:

Hijama for the prostate is a type of Hijama that is applied to sites associated to the prostate, urinary system, and male reproductive system, such as the lower belly, lower back, and inner ankle. The prostate is a walnut-sized gland that generates and secretes fluid to nourish and protect sperm. It is placed beneath the bladder and encircles the urethra. Several disorders can affect the prostate, including inflammation, infection, enlargement, and malignancy. Hijama for the prostate can have various benefits, including:

Improving Prostate Function and Health

Hijama for the prostate can help to improve prostate function and health by stimulating the prostate and epididymis. It can also balance testosterone and estrogen levels and help prevent or cure illnesses like benign prostatic hyperplasia (BPH), prostatitis, and prostate cancer. The points for this benefit are the lower abdomen, navel, stomach, and spleen.

Improving the urine and sexual function

Hijama for the prostate can improve urinary and sexual function by increasing blood circulation and oxygenation to the bladder, urethra, and penis. It can also help with symptoms of urinary tract infections (UTIs), urine incontinence, erectile dysfunction, and premature ejaculation. This advantage is provided by spots on the chest, neck, upper and lower lungs, and upper back.

Hijama for Inflammatory joint rheumatism:

Hijama for inflammatory joint rheumatism is a type of Hijama that is applied to sites associated to the joints, muscles, and immune system, such as the lower back, hip, and shoulder. Inflammatory joint rheumatism refers to a variety of disorders that cause joint inflammation, pain, and stiffness, including rheumatoid arthritis, gout, and lupus. Hijama for inflammatory joint rheumatism can have various benefits, including:

Relieving pain and inflammation

Hijama for inflammatory joint rheumatism can help with pain and inflammation by relieving pressure and swelling in the joints and nerves. It can also regulate the hormones and neurotransmitters that influence pain perception and inflammation. The points for this benefit include the lower back, hips, knees, and shoulders.

Improving Joint Mobility and Posture

Hijama for inflammatory joint rheumatism can help with joint mobility and posture by relaxing the muscles and tendons that support the joints. It can also help to prevent or treat diseases like scoliosis, kyphosis, and lordosis, which impact the curvature of the spine. This advantage is available in the lower back, middle back, upper back, and neck locations.

Stimulating Healing and Recovery

Hijama for inflammatory joint rheumatism can help with healing and recovery by boosting the immune system and defending against infections and diseases. It can also help in the regeneration and repair of damaged tissues and organs. This advantage is provided by areas on the upper back, liver, spleen, and lower back.

Hijama Cupping therapy for gynecological diseases and menstrual pain:

Hijama for gynecological illnesses and menstrual discomfort is a type of Hijama that targets reproductive, hormonal, and fertility areas such as the lower belly, lower back, and inner ankle. Gynecological diseases are conditions that affect the female reproductive organs, which include the uterus, ovaries, fallopian tubes, vagina, and breast. Common gynecological illnesses include menstruation abnormalities, pelvic inflammatory disease, endometriosis, fibroids, and ovarian cysts. Menstrual discomfort, also known as dysmenorrhea, refers to pain or cramps that occur before or during the menstrual cycle. Hijama for gynecological illnesses and menstrual pain can have various benefits, including:

Improving menstrual cycle and fertility.

Hijama for gynecological problems and menstrual discomfort can help with menstrual cycle and fertility by stimulating the ovaries and uterus. It can also control hormones and the menstrual cycle, helping to prevent or cure disorders like amenorrhea, oligomenorrhea, menorrhagia, and polycystic ovary syndrome. The points for this benefit are the lower abdomen, navel, stomach, and spleen.

Relieving menstruation pain and cramping

Hijama for gynecological illnesses and menstruation pain might reduce menstrual pain and cramps by improving blood flow and oxygen to the pelvic region. It can also calm muscles and nerves, reducing inflammation and spasms. This advantage is provided by spots on the chest, neck, upper and lower lungs, and upper back.

Balancing the mood and emotions

Hijama for gynecological problems and monthly discomfort help regulate mood and emotions by activating the pineal gland and melatonin. It can also regulate mood and hormones, reducing stress, anxiety, and sadness. This advantage is provided by the locations on the top of the head, forehead, heart, and inner wrists.

Hijama Cupping therapy for anti-aging:

Hijama for anti-aging is a type of Hijama that focuses on skin, blood, and vitality spots such as the upper back, forehead, and lower back. Anti-aging is the act of postponing or reversing the effects of aging, such as wrinkles, sagging skin, age spots, and hair loss. Hijama can offer a variety of anti-aging advantages, including:

Cleansing the skin and blood

Hijama for anti-aging can cleanse the skin and blood by removing toxins and waste from the body and psyche. It can also enhance complexion and vision, as well as treat skin conditions like acne, eczema, psoriasis, and infections. This advantage is available at the upper back, liver, kidney, and lower back sites.

Stimulating collagen and elastin

Hijama for anti-aging can stimulate collagen and elastin by creating negative pressure within the cups. This may improve oxygen intake and blood flow to the skin and tissues. The points for this benefit include the forehead, between the brows, nasal bridge, and cheek points.

Boosting energy and vitality

Hijama for anti-aging can improve energy and vitality by increasing blood flow and oxygen to the brain and body. It can also purge the mind of bad thoughts and emotions, boosting awareness and intuition. The points for this benefit are at the top of the head, the forehead, between the brows, and on the nose bridge.

Menopause and Hijama:

Menopause and Hijama is a sort of Hijama that focuses on locations associated with the hormonal system, reproductive system, and sleep, such as the lower belly, lower back, and forehead. Menopause is the normal stage of a woman's life in which her ovaries stop producing eggs and her menstrual cycles halt. It often develops between the ages of 45 and 55 and is accompanied by a variety of physical and emotional symptoms, including hot flashes, nocturnal sweats, mood swings, sleeplessness, and vaginal dryness. Hijama for menopause can provide a variety of benefits, including:

Balancing hormones and emotions

Hijama for menopause can regulate hormones and emotions by activating the pineal gland and melatonin. It can also regulate estrogen and progesterone levels, reducing stress, anxiety, and depression. This advantage is provided by the locations on the top of the head, forehead, heart, and inner wrists.

Relieving hot flashes and nocturnal sweats

Hijama for menopause can help decrease hot flashes and night sweats by lowering heat and congestion in the body and brain. It can also control body temperature and sweat glands, preventing or treating illnesses including fever, infection, and dehydration. This advantage is provided by spots on the chest, neck, upper and lower lungs, and upper back.

Enhancing sleep and relaxation

Hijama for menopause can improve sleep and relaxation by stimulating the vagus nerve and the parasympathetic nervous system. It can also help to regulate the circadian rhythm and sleep cycle, as well as cure insomnia and other sleep disorders. This advantage is provided by the locations on the top of the head, forehead, heart, and inner wrists.

Hijama for test excitement and attention deficit:

Hijama for test excitement and attention deficit is a sort of Hijama that focuses on the brain, neurological system, and mental health, such as the top of the head, forehead, and back of the head. Test excitement and attention deficit are circumstances that impair the capacity to focus, concentrate, and perform well on exams or other tasks. Test excitement can generate anxiety, anxiousness, and stress, while attention deficiency can create distraction, impulsivity, and hyperactivity. Hijama for test excitement and attention deficit can provide various benefits, including:

Improving memory and recall

Hijama for test excitement and attention deficit can boost memory and recall by increasing blood flow and oxygen to the brain and body. It can also purge the mind of bad thoughts and emotions, boosting awareness and intuition. The points for this benefit are at the top of the head, the forehead, between the brows, and on the nose bridge.

Enhancing cognitive and creative abilities

Hijama for test excitement and attention deficit can improve cognitive and creative skills by engaging the brain's right and left hemispheres, as well as their integration and balance. It can also improve verbal and nonverbal communication skills, as well as interpersonal interactions. This advantage is available through the following points: back of the head, shoulder, side of the neck, and front of the neck.

Calming emotions and nerves

Hijama can help with test anxiety and attention deficit by activating the vagus nerve and the parasympathetic nervous system. It can also regulate mood and hormones, reducing stress, anxiety, and sadness. This advantage is provided by the locations on the top of the head, forehead, heart, and inner wrists.

Hijama cupping therapy for Diabetes:

Hijama for diabetes is a type of Hijama that is applied to areas connected to the pancreas, blood sugar, and metabolism, such as the lower belly, lower back, and inner ankle. Diabetes is a condition in which the body is unable to generate or use insulin adequately, resulting in excessive blood sugar levels and other consequences. Hijama for diabetes can have various benefits, including:

Improving insulin production and sensitivity

Hijama for diabetes can boost insulin production and sensitivity by stimulating the pancreatic and liver. It can also control blood sugar levels and help prevent or cure illnesses like type 1, type 2, and gestational diabetes. The points for this benefit are the lower abdomen, navel, stomach, and spleen.

Enhancing blood circulation and oxygenation

Hijama for diabetes can improve blood circulation and oxygenation by producing negative pressure within the cups. This may boost oxygen intake and blood flow to the organs and tissues. This advantage is provided by spots on the chest, neck, upper and lower lungs, and upper back.

Stimulating Healing and Recovery

Hijama for diabetes can help with healing and recovery by boosting the immune system and resistance against infections and diseases. It can also help in the regeneration and repair of damaged tissues and organs. The lower back points, liver point, kidney point, and upper back points are the points for this benefit.

Hijama cupping therapy for athletes:

Hijama for athletes is a sort of Hijama that focuses on locations associated to muscles, joints, and performance, such as the lower back, hip, and shoulder. Athletes are susceptible to a variety of ailments, pain, and stress, which can impair their physical and mental performance. Hijama for athletes can have a variety of benefits, including:

decreasing pain and inflammation

Hijama for athletes can help with pain and inflammation by lowering pressure and swelling in the muscles and nerves. It can also regulate the hormones and neurotransmitters that influence pain perception and inflammation. The points for this benefit include the lower back, hips, knees, and shoulders.

Improving Joint Mobility and Posture

Hijama for athletes can help with joint mobility and posture by relaxing the muscles and tendons that support the joints. It can also help to prevent or treat diseases like scoliosis, kyphosis, and lordosis, which impact the curvature of the spine. This advantage is available in the lower back, middle back, upper back, and neck locations.

Boosting energy and vitality

Hijama for athletes can boost energy and vitality by increasing blood flow and oxygen to the brain and body. It can also purge the mind of bad thoughts and emotions, boosting awareness and intuition. The points for this benefit are at the top of the head, the forehead, between the brows, and on the nose bridge.

Hijama cupping therapy in Children:

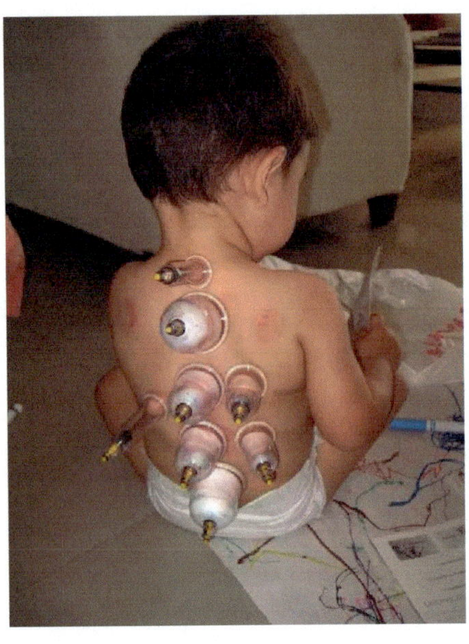

Hijama in children is a type of Hijama that is applied to areas relevant to growth, development, and immunity, such as the upper back, forehead, and lower back. Children are susceptible to a variety of illnesses and infections, which can have an impact on both their physical and mental health. Hijama in children can offer a variety of benefits, including:

Improving the immune system and protection

Hijama in children can help to enhance their immune system and defense by eliminating toxins and waste from their bodies and minds. It can also enhance complexion and vision, as well as treat skin conditions like acne, eczema, psoriasis, and infections. This advantage is available at the upper back, liver, kidney, and lower back sites.

Promoting growth and development

Hijama in children can promote growth and development by activating the pituitary gland and growth hormone. It can also regulate hormones and development factors, preventing or treating diseases like dwarfism, gigantism, and delayed puberty. The points for this benefit are at the top of the head, the forehead, between the brows, and on the nose bridge.

Improving learning and concentration

Hijama can help youngsters learn and concentrate better by stimulating the right and left hemispheres of the brain and promoting their integration and balance. It can also improve verbal and nonverbal communication skills, as well as interpersonal interactions. This advantage is available through the following points: back of the head, shoulder, side of the neck, and front of the neck.

Hijama cupping therapy for varicose veins:

Hijama for varicose veins is a type of Hijama that is applied to vein, blood, and circulation-related locations such as the lower leg, lower back, and chest. Varicose veins are twisted, enlarged, or swollen veins that appear beneath the skin. They are produced by high blood pressure in the veins, which can be caused by a variety of reasons including prolonged standing or sitting, pregnancy, obesity, or a hereditary predisposition. Hijama for varicose veins can offer various benefits, including:

Lowering blood pressure and cholesterol levels

Hijama for varicose veins helps lower blood pressure and cholesterol by reducing blood volume and viscosity. It can also balance the hormones and neurotransmitters that control blood pressure and inflammation. This advantage applies to the chest, upper back, liver, and lower back locations.

Relaxing the veins and muscles

Hijama for varicose veins helps relax the veins and the muscles by creating a negative pressure inside the cups. This can help to increase joint and limb flexibility. The points for this benefit include the inner ankle, lower leg, knee, and hip.

Cleaning the Blood and Skin

Hijama for varicose veins helps cleanse the blood and skin by eliminating toxins and wastes from the body and psyche. It can also enhance complexion and vision, as well as treat skin conditions like acne, eczema, psoriasis, and infections. This advantage is available at the upper back, liver, kidney, and lower back sites.

Hijama for hormonal complications:

Hijama for hormonal disorders is a type of Hijama that focuses on locations associated with the hormone system, reproductive system, and mood, such as the lower belly, lower back, and forehead. Hormonal issues are conditions that disrupt the balance and function of hormones, which are chemical messengers that regulate a variety of bodily processes such as growth, metabolism, reproduction, and mood. Stress, illness, medication, and disease are all potential causes of hormonal disorders. Hijama for hormone issues can have various benefits, including:

Balancing hormones and emotions

Hijama for hormonal disorders can regulate hormones and emotions by activating the pineal gland and melatonin. It can help balance the levels of estrogen and progesterone in women, as well as testosterone in men. It can also help with stress, anxiety, and depression. This advantage is provided by the locations on the top of the head, forehead, heart, and inner wrists.

Improving reproductive and sexual functions

Hijama for hormonal disorders can help with reproductive and sexual function by stimulating the ovaries and uterus in women and the testicles and prostate in males. It can help control the menstrual cycle and fertility in women, as well as the quality of sperm and libido in males. The points for this benefit are the lower abdomen, navel, stomach, and spleen.

Improving the metabolism and digestion

Hijama for hormonal disorders can help with metabolism and digestion by stimulating the thyroid and pancreas. It can also help to balance blood sugar and weight, as well as prevent or cure illnesses including diabetes, obesity, and thyroid disorders. The points for this benefit are the lower abdomen, navel, stomach, and spleen.

Chapter
07

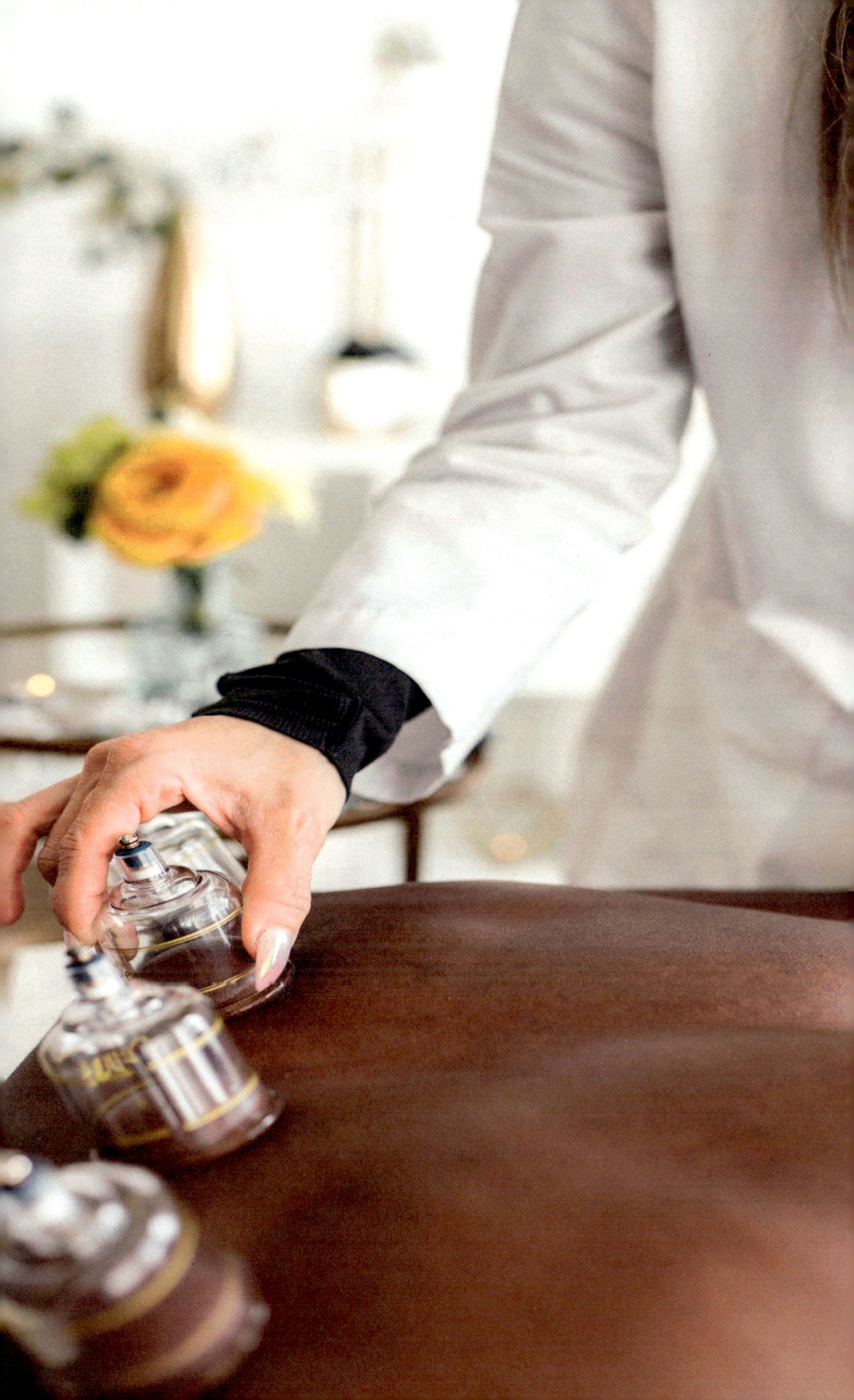

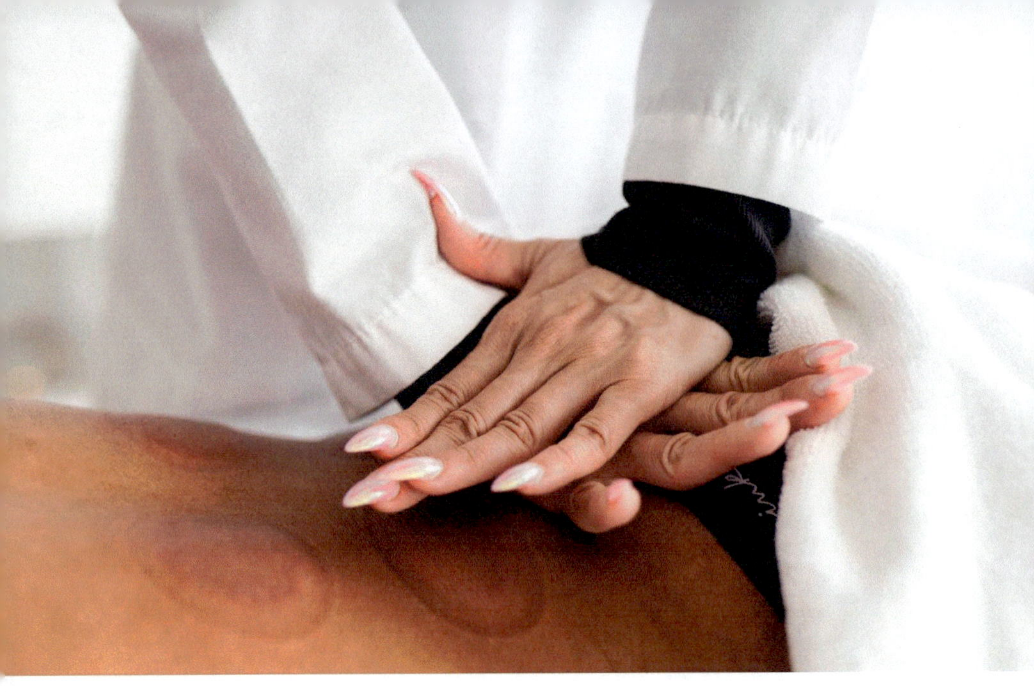

Risks and Precautions of Hijama Cupping Therapy

What Are the risks and Safety precautions for Hijama Cupping Therapy?

Hijama cupping therapy has numerous benefits and impacts, including improving the nervous system, endocrine system, blood circulation, immune system, and lymphatic system. It can also be used to prevent and cure a variety of diseases and conditions, including diabetes, pain, hypertension, arthritis, asthma, skin problems, infertility, and others. Nonetheless, there are certain potential hazards and side effects linked with Hijama cupping therapy, such as infection, bleeding, bruising, scarring, anemia, fainting, and so on. Thus, it is vital to understand the dangers and safety precautions related with Hijama cupping therapy, as well as to follow specific guidelines and suggestions for decreasing and managing such risks and side effects. These include checking the patient's medical history and vital signs, avoiding specific areas and spots, following the suggested time and frequency, keeping a watch out for both general and specific contraindications, and seeking medical attention as needed. This chapter will give you more information about the potential hazards and safety precautions linked with Hijama cupping therapy, as well as practical recommendations for executing the therapy.

The possible risks and some side effects of Hijama cupping therapy

Hijama cupping therapy removes blood and toxins from the underlying tissues by tiny skin incisions and suction cups. This process has the potential to cause bleeding, bruising, infection, scarring, anemia, fainting, and other complications. These dangers and side effects may have an impact on the patient's health and well-being, and their likelihood and severity might vary depending on a number of factors, such as the practitioner's training and experience, the quality and cleanliness of the equipment, the patient's condition and constitution, and so on. As a result, it is vital to recognize, assess, and appreciate the potential risks and side effects of Hijama cupping therapy, as well as their causes and consequences. The following are some potential risks and side effects of Hijama cupping therapy:

Virus Infection

A bacterial, viral, or fungal infection is when germs invade and proliferate in the body, causing discomfort, fever, pus, or inflammation. Infections can occur during or after Hijama cupping therapy if the patient's immune system is impaired or has an existing infection, the wounds are not properly cleaned and treated, or the equipment is not thoroughly sanitized. The area of the body where the Hijama cupping therapy was administered may get infected, or it may spread to other locations such as the blood, bones, joints, or organs. If an infection is not treated promptly and properly, it might result in serious complications such as organ failure, arthritis, sepsis, or osteomyelitis. To prevent and cure infection, it is vital to use sterile equipment, clean and dress wounds, and take antibiotics as prescribed.

Bleeding

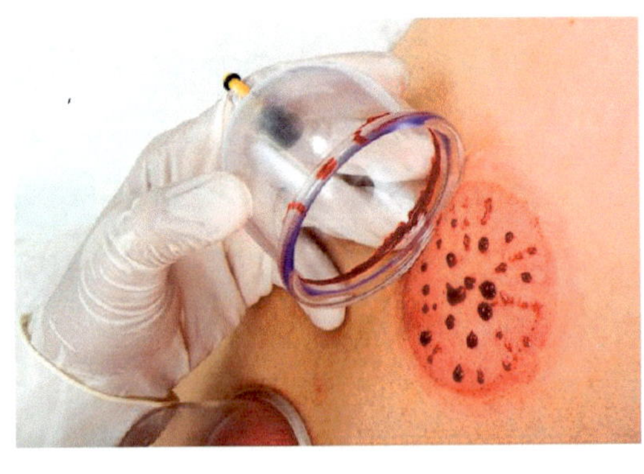

The loss of blood from the body, known as bleeding, can cause shock, weariness, or disorientation. If the patient has a bleeding disorder or is taking blood thinners, bleeding may occur during or after Hijama cupping therapy, especially if the incisions are made too deeply or repeatedly, or if the suction is performed too vigorously or for too long. The local area where the Hijama cupping therapy was provided may have been affected by bleeding, as well as blood loss and anemia, a condition characterized by a low concentration of red blood cells or hemoglobin, which can worsen weakness, weariness, and dyspnea. Bleeding can also generate blood clots, which are blood clumps that can restrict blood vessels and, if they reach the brain, heart, or lungs, cause a stroke, heart attack, or pulmonary embolism. As a result, it is vital to stop bleeding and apply pressure as needed, in addition to making small, shallow incisions and applying moderate to vigorous suction.

bruising

Bruising may cause discomfort, stiffness, or irritation. It is the redness and swelling of the skin caused by the rupture of blood vessels under the surface. Bruising may occur during or after Hijama cupping therapy if the patient is using blood thinners, has delicate or sensitive skin, the suction is too strong or prolonged, or the

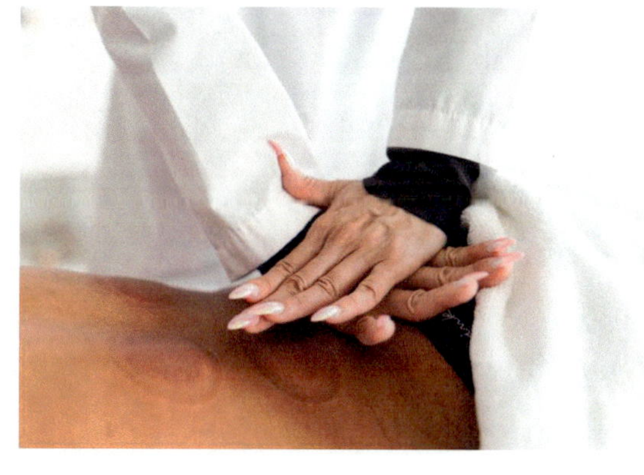

cups are changed or removed too rapidly. Bruising may cause cosmetic or aesthetic problems, such as unsightly skin lines or blotches, or it may affect the area surrounding the Hijama cupping therapy technique. Bruising can also have functional consequences, such as restricted movement or decreased feeling in the affected area. As a result, it is necessary to prevent and treat bruising by using ice or cold compresses to the affected area, slowly withdrawing the cups with moderate suction, and so on.

Scarring

Scarring is the process by which fibrous tissue replaces normal skin following an injury. This can lead to functional or cosmetic problems such contracture, keloid, or deformity. Scarring may happen from Hijama cupping therapy if the patient has a slow or poor healing process, a genetic predisposition to scarring, too many or too deep incisions, inadequate wound care, or none at all. Scarring can cause irregular or raised scars, changes in the color or texture of the skin, and problems with appearance or cosmetics that can harm the area where the Hijama cupping therapy was applied locally. Scarring can cause functional

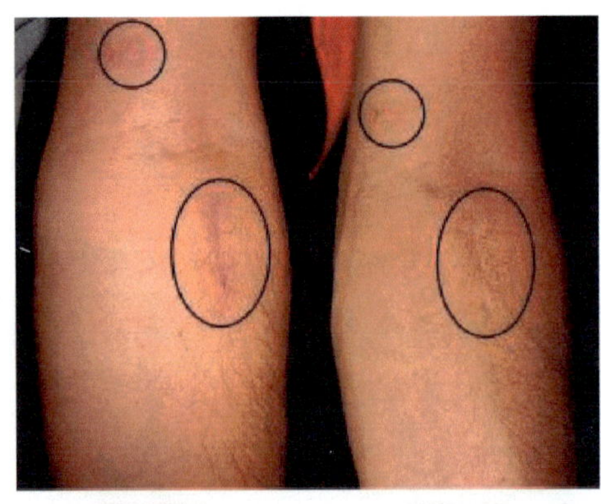

concerns such as reduced skin elasticity or movement, as well as increased discomfort or sensitivity in the affected area. As a result, it is vital to prevent and treat scarring by applying moisturizers or scar therapies to the afflicted area, cleaning and treating wounds, and making small, shallow incisions.

Anemia

Anemia is defined as a low concentration of red blood cells, or hemoglobin, which can cause weakness, tiredness, and shortness of breath. Hijama cupping therapy may cause anemia if the patient has insufficient or inadequate synthesis of red blood cells or hemoglobin, such as iron deficiency, vitamin B12 deficiency, or sickle cell anemia, or if blood loss is significant or frequent. Anemia can cause specific symptoms such as pale skin, cold hands and feet, a rapid heartbeat, headaches, or chest pain, or it can affect the entire body. Anemia can cause heart failure, arrhythmia, or stroke if oxygen is not delivered to the organs and tissues in sufficient quantities. Thus, it is crucial to prevent and treat anemia by limiting the amount and frequency of blood loss, monitoring the patient's iron and hemoglobin levels, and providing iron supplements or blood transfusions as needed.

Losing consciousness

A drop in blood pressure or blood flow to the brain can cause a person to faint, which is a momentary loss of consciousness that might result in injury, confusion, or drowsiness. Patients who are exhausted, anxious, or have low blood pressure, cardiac difficulties, or neurological concerns may experience fainting during or after Hijama cupping therapy. Fainting can have a full-body affect or specialized symptoms such as dizziness, nausea, sweating, or impaired vision. If the patient loses equilibrium or collides with something while fainting, it can lead to fractures, falls, or head injuries. As a result, it is vital to prevent and manage fainting by keeping the patient adequately fed, hydrated, and rested; monitoring the patient's blood pressure and pulse; and, if the patient feels faint, placing them on their side and lifting their legs.

Hijama cupping therapy rules and recommendations for reducing and monitoring risks and negative effects

Hijama cupping therapy is an alternative medical technique that uses cups to generate a vacuum on the skin, extracting toxins and blood from the tissues beneath it. Hijama cupping therapy has numerous benefits and impacts, including improving the nervous system, endocrine system, blood circulation, immune system, and lymphatic system. It can also be used to prevent and cure a variety of diseases and conditions, including diabetes, pain, hypertension, arthritis, asthma, skin problems, infertility, and others. Nonetheless, there are certain potential hazards and side effects linked with Hijama cupping therapy, such as infection, bleeding, bruising, scarring, anemia, fainting, and so on.

Thus, it is vital to understand the dangers and safety precautions related with Hijama cupping therapy, as well as to follow specific guidelines and suggestions for decreasing and managing such risks and side effects. These include checking the patient's medical history and vital signs, avoiding specific areas and spots, following the suggested time and frequency, keeping a watch out for both general and specific contraindications, and seeking medical attention as needed. This section will offer you with further information on how to properly and successfully do Hijama cupping therapy, as well as instructions and recommendations for decreasing and regulating the procedure's dangers and bad effects.

Examining the patient's medical history and vital signs:

Before beginning Hijama cupping therapy, you should check the patient's medical history and ensure that all of their vital signs—including blood pressure, pulse, temperature, and blood sugar—remain stable and normal. In addition, you should inquire about any allergies, prescription drugs, illnesses, or difficulties the patient may have that could affect the course of treatment, such as infections, bleeding disorders, diabetes, hypertension, and so on. By analyzing the patient's medical history and vital signs, you may decide whether they are a good candidate for Hijama cupping therapy and help avoid any unwanted or unpleasant reactions. To ensure the treatment's safety and efficacy, as well as to personalize it to the patient's needs and preferences, you should also evaluate the patient's vital signs and medical record. You can use a range of techniques and devices to confirm the patient's vital signs and medical history, including:

- Asking that the patient fill out a consent form or questionnaire containing questions about their personal information, past medical history, current medications, allergies, symptoms, complaints, expectations, and other details.

- Using a stethoscope, sphygmomanometer, thermometer, and glucometer, monitor the patient's blood pressure, pulse, temperature, and blood sugar levels and compare the results to the standard ranges and values.

- Keep an eye out for signs of disease, distress, or discomfort, such as pale skin, cold hands and feet, a fast heartbeat, chest pain, or a headache, as well as the patient's behavior, emotional state, and physical look.

Preventing particular areas and points on the body:

When utilizing Hijama cupping therapy, avoid using the cups to body parts such as the eyes, ears, nose, mouth, genitalia, nipples, moles, wounds, or inflamed or infected areas because they may cause pain or discomfort to the patient. Acupoints such as Ren-1 (Huiyin), which may induce labor, and GB-21 (Jianjing), which may cause fainting, should not be treated with cups since the effects may be adverse. Staying away from specified sites and regions reduces the risk of hurting sensitive or critical organs or tissues, as well as any disruption or inconsistency with regular physiological processes or functions. You can respect the patient's privacy and dignity while also helping them avoid pain, discomfort, or shame by avoiding specified areas and sites. To avoid specific areas and spots, you can use a variety of approaches and tools, such as those listed below:

- Using a diagram or chart to illustrate the locations and functions of the body's many points and sites, as well as which ones should be avoided or used with caution.

- Make a note of the locations and spots where you wish to apply the cups with a marker or pen, and avoid going anywhere that is hazardous or unsuitable for Hijama cupping therapy.

- Using your expertise and experience, you should be able to identify places and spots that potentially harm or disturb the patient and either avoid them or use them sparingly.

Consider the right time and frequency:

During Hijama cupping therapy, you should adhere to the appropriate timing and frequency of the therapy, which will optimize the benefits and prevent issues. You should consider all elements that may influence the timing and frequency, such as the patient's age, gender, health, and constitution; the season, temperature, and lunar phase; the type, style, and purpose of Hijama cupping therapy; and so on. By following the specified schedule and frequency, you may minimize the risks and side effects of Hijama cupping therapy, such as infection, bleeding, bruising, scars, anemia, fainting, and so on, while simultaneously maximizing its benefits and outcomes. Aside from assisting you in harmonizing the therapy with cosmic and environmental influences and energies, using the proper time and frequency will also help you match the treatment with the body's natural and physiological cycles and rhythms. To maintain the proper timing and frequency, you can use a variety of techniques and instruments, such as the ones listed below:

- Use a planner or calendar to display the treatment dates and times, as well as the best and worst times to receive Hijama cupping therapy based on the lunar phase, season, and weather. For example, Hijama cupping therapy should be performed on the full moon days, which are the 17th, 19th, and 21st of the lunar month.

- Using a stopwatch or timer, measure the length of time and intervals between treatments, ensuring that the bleeding and suction are not overly long or short, and that the recovery and rest are not overly long or short. For example, depending on the patient's health and constitution, Hijama cupping therapy should be performed for 10 to 15 minutes every session and repeated every 2 to 4 weeks.

- Using your knowledge and experience, determine the best time and frequency of treatment for the patient depending on age, gender, health, constitution, and the type, mode, and purpose of Hijama cupping therapy. For example, it is recommended that young, healthy patients receive Hijama cupping therapy more frequently and with less intensity, whereas elderly and sick patients receive it less frequently and with greater intensity.

Taking careful note of general and particular contraindications:

You should be informed of the general and specific contraindications of Hijama cupping therapy before, during, and after the procedure. These may indicate that the patient is not an ideal candidate for the treatment, that it should be discontinued, or that it should be modified. You should consider any variables that may indicate a contraindication, such as the patient's symptoms, signs, or complaints; the appearance, color, or volume of the blood; the patient's response or feedback, and so on. By following the general and individual contraindications, you can assist prevent harm or damage to the patient while also avoiding interference or contradiction with the therapy. Following the general and specific contraindications allows you to respect the patient's wants and choices while also assuring their safety and comfort. You can use a variety of ways and resources to keep track of the general and specific contraindications, including:

- Hijama cupping therapy should be avoided if a patient has any of the conditions stated on a checklist or form. The patient must confirm or deny their presence or absence prior to, during, and following the treatment. Women who are pregnant or have their periods, children or the elderly, people who are weak or disabled, people who have severe or acute diseases or conditions, people who have skin or blood disorders, people who are fasting or have eaten too much, and so on should not receive Hijama cupping therapy.

- You can use a scale or meter to assess the severity of the patient's symptoms, signs, or complaints, and then compare them to what is regarded normal or acceptable before, during, and after treatment. Patients with high or low blood pressure, blood sugar, hemoglobin, or fever should avoid Hijama cupping treatment.

- To decide whether to continue, stop, or change the treatment depending on the blood's appearance, color, or quantity, as well as the patient's response or feedback. For example, if the patient is pale, chilly, or feeble, suggesting a loss of blood or energy, or if the blood is dark, thick, or clotted, indicating the presence of taiba or impurities, Hijama cupping therapy should be discontinued or modified.

Getting medical help if necessary

Following Hijama cupping therapy, you should monitor the patient and follow up to ensure they are healing and progressing as predicted. Furthermore, if the patient experiences any severe or persistent symptoms or complications—such as fever, infection, bleeding, anemia, fainting, and so on—you should advise them to seek medical attention. If necessary, seeking medical attention can assist you in ensuring that the patient obtains the proper diagnosis and treatment for any symptoms or repercussions, as well as preventing the patient from experiencing further injury. If necessary, seeking medical attention can also assist you avoid legal or ethical ramifications, as well as respect the Hijama cupping treatment profession's standards and responsibilities. If necessary, you can receive medical care via a variety of approaches and services, such as:

- Calling an emergency service, such as 911 or 119, and notifying them about the patient's condition and situation, in addition to requesting medical advice or assistance. This can be accomplished through a computer or telephone contact to the patient's primary care physician.

- Giving a patient basic or emergency care with a first aid or medical kit. This treatment may include cleaning and treating wounds, applying pressure to stop bleeding, delivering oxygen or doing CPR to restore breathing, and other duties.

- Making decisions regarding whether to continue, discontinue, or modify therapy, or to refer the patient to a medical specialist or a hospital, necessitates using your knowledge and experience to recognize and assess the severity and urgency of symptoms or complications.

Chapter
08

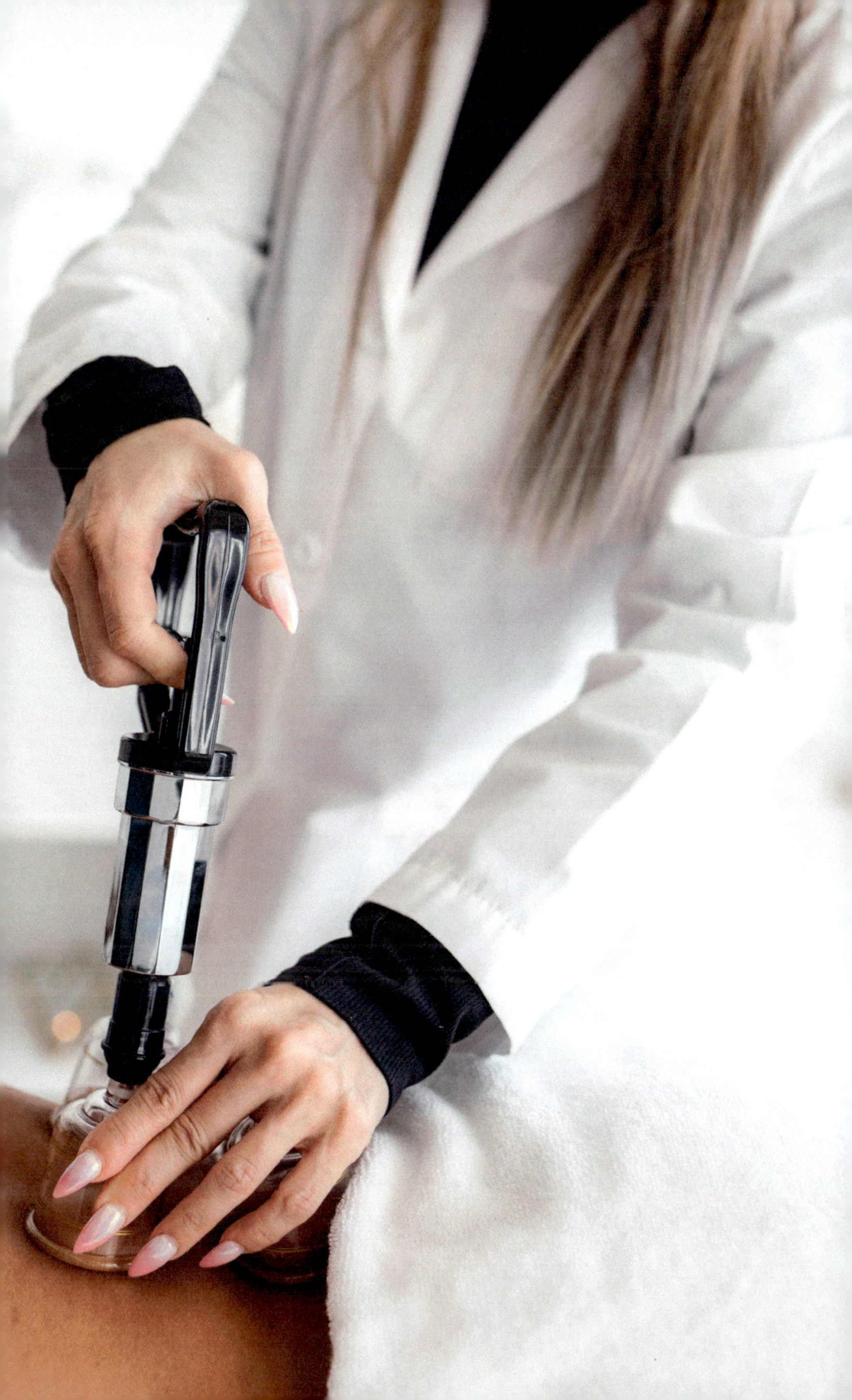

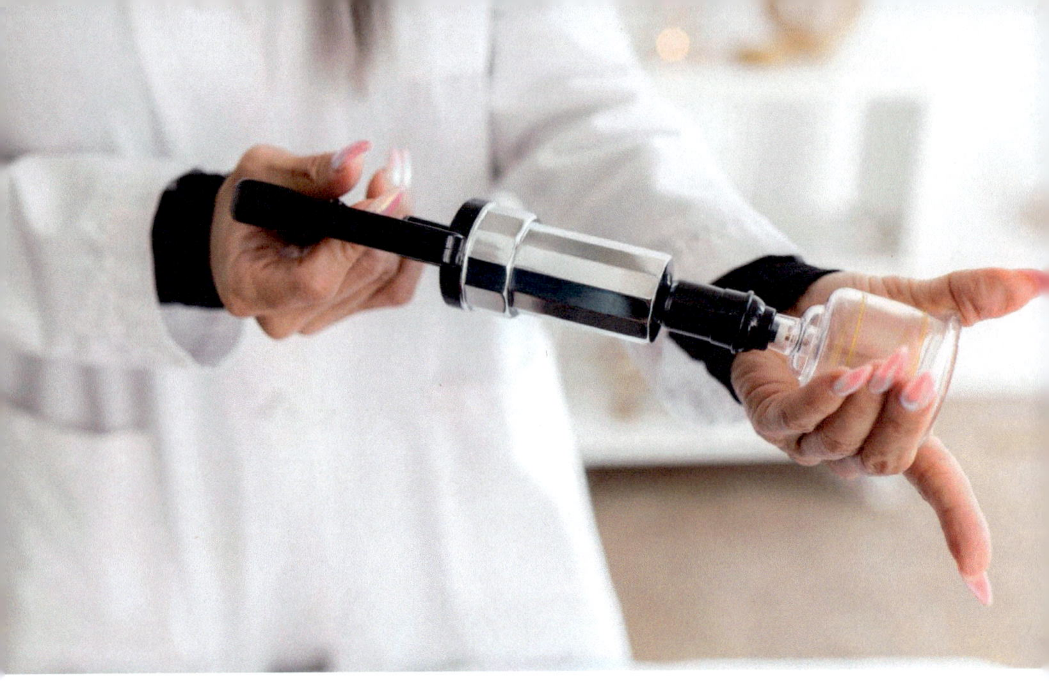

Future Trends in Cupping Therapy

What Are the Future Trends in Cupping Therapy?

Cupping therapy has grown in popularity and notoriety in recent years, particularly as celebrities and athletes have expressed interest in and endorsement of the procedure. Cupping therapy has also been combined with other techniques, such as acupuncture, massage, and herbal medicine, to increase and supplement their respective effects and advantages. Cupping therapy has also been improved with new technology, such as smart cups and digital pumps, to increase its convenience and efficiency. Cupping therapy has also been investigated and evidenced using innovative methodologies such as randomized controlled trials, meta-analyses, and so on to confirm and verify the technique's efficacy and safety.

This chapter will teach you about the future trends in cupping therapy, such as its integration, innovation, and research, as well as the problems and possibilities that it will encounter in the future.

The advancement of cupping therapy with new technologies

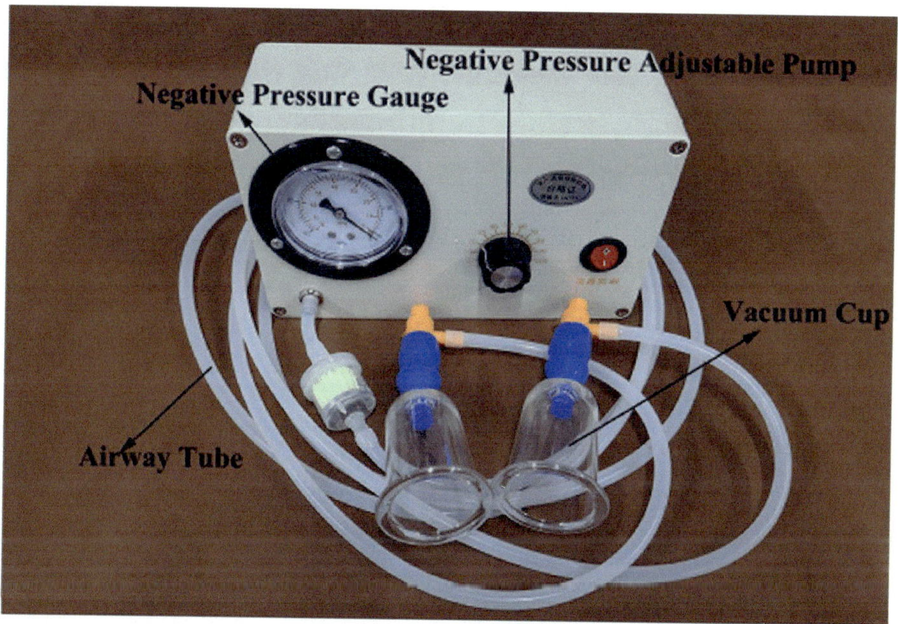

Another potential trend in cupping therapy is the use of new technology like smart cups and digital pumps. Cupping therapy innovation with new technologies has the potential to improve and modernize the quality and convenience of cupping therapy by adding more features and functions to the cups, as well as making the cups more user-friendly. The use of modern technologies in cupping therapy can create new opportunities and problems for practitioners and patients, who can explore and experiment with the cups and benefit or suffer from them.

There is some evidence and instances of the benefits and drawbacks of combining cupping therapy with new technologies, from both practical and theoretical perspectives. However, further study and assessment are required to analyze the impact and implications of cupping therapy innovation using new technology, as well as to compare it to other interventions, such as traditional cupping therapy or no intervention. Cupping therapy has the potential to revolutionize the following technologies:

Smart cups

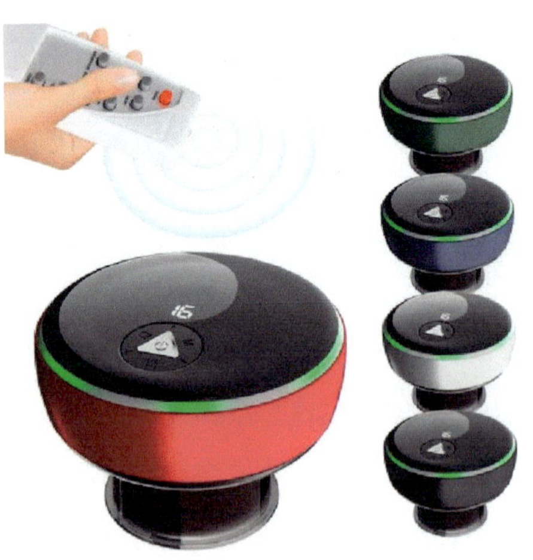

Smart cups are a type of cup that has been fitted with sensors, chips, or displays. These devices can measure and track different parameters, including the pressure, temperature, duration, and frequency of the cup. Additionally, they can communicate and work together with other devices through wireless or Bluetooth connections, such as computers, tablets, and smartphones. By enabling more customization and personalization, offering more accurate and precise control and feedback, and storing and sharing the data and information of the cups, smart cups can enhance and modernize the quality and ease of cupping therapy. Some of the advantages of smart cups are:

- They provide real-time and historical data and information about the cups, including their pressure, temperature, duration, and frequency. They can also recommend the optimal settings and modes based on the algorithms and models of the cups, assisting practitioners and patients in customizing and optimizing the cups to their needs, preferences, and conditions.

- Through the tracking and recording of changes and effects, such as blood flow, skin color, pain level, and patient satisfaction, they can assist practitioners and patients in monitoring and evaluating the cups. Additionally, they can provide feedback and reports on the cups based on the analysis and interpretation of the cups.

- By permitting remote and wireless control and access to the cups—such as turning them on and off, adjusting their temperature and pressure, and setting timers and alarms—as well as the sharing and exchange of data and information about the cups—such as sending and receiving data and information, comparing and reviewing the data and information—they can facilitate communication between the patients and practitioners.

Digital pumps

Digital pumps are those that run on electricity or batteries, have the ability to create and modify the suction in the cups, and can be integrated into the valves or cups via buttons or switches, or they can be connected to them via tubes or wires. By offering 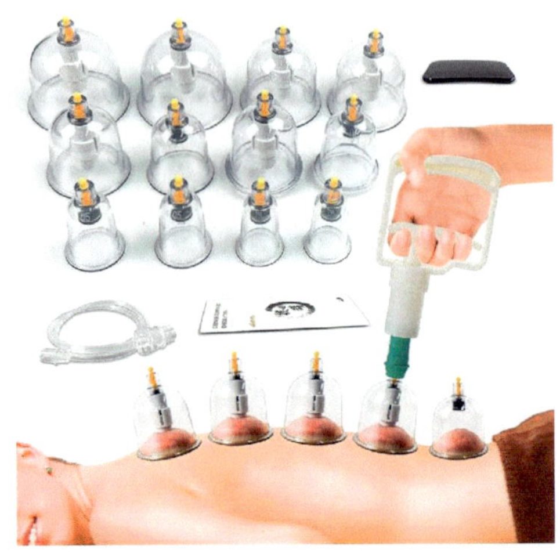 more consistent and dependable cup suction, increasing cup flexibility and variety, and lowering the risk and inconvenience of cup leaks, noise, or fire, digital pumps can enhance and modernize the quality and ease of cupping therapy.

The following are a few benefits of digital pumps:

- By producing and controlling the vacuum of the cups, avoiding the use of fire, air, or water to create the suction of the cups, and preventing the loss of suction due to air leakage or pressure changes in the cups, they can assist practitioners and patients in creating and maintaining the suction of the cups.

- They can facilitate the use of various cup sizes and types, such as glass, plastic, or silicone cups, as well as small, medium, and large cups. They can also facilitate the application of various cup methods and techniques, such as moving, stationary, or flash cups. All of these features can assist practitioners and patients in adjusting and varying the suction of the cups.

- In addition to lowering and preventing the occurrence of fire, noise, or leakage of the cups, they can assist practitioners and patients in minimizing and reducing the risk and inconvenience associated with the cups. This includes minimizing or eliminating the use of fire, air, or water to create the suction of the cups, as well as reducing and minimizing damage and injury associated with the cups, such as burns, blisters, or bruises.

The integration of cupping therapy with other modalities

The fusion of cupping therapy with other modalities, such acupuncture, massage, herbal medicine, etc., is one of the emerging concepts in cupping therapy. By operating on several levels and parts of the body, including the physical, energetic, emotional, and mental levels, the combination of cupping therapy with other modalities can augment and complete their effects and advantages. When cupping treatment is combined with other modalities, it can give practitioners and patients additional options and flexibility. They can decide which combination and application of cupping therapy with other modalities best suits their requirements, preferences, and conditions.

From both the traditional and contemporary viewpoints, there is some proof and instances of the safety and efficacy of combining cupping therapy with other techniques. To determine the best and most consistent methods and procedures for the fusion of cupping therapy with other modalities, additional study and standards are still required. The following are a few methods that can be combined with cupping therapy:

The use of acupuncture

Using tiny needles inserted into predetermined body sites known as acupoints, acupuncture is an ancient Chinese medical practice that aims to balance the opposing forces of yin and yang and promote the flow of qi, or life energy. By applying the cups to the same or nearby acupoints as the needles, or by inserting the needles after removing the cups, cupping therapy can be combined with acupuncture to improve qi stimulation and regulation and treat or prevent a variety of illnesses and conditions, including pain, inflammation, infection, and so forth.

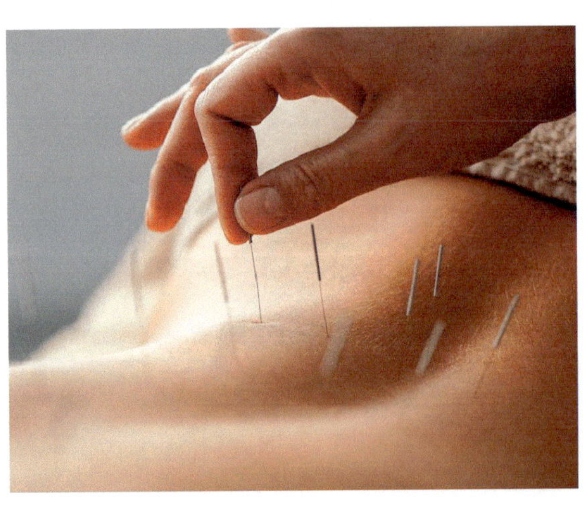

According to the tenets of traditional Chinese medicine, the combination of cupping therapy and acupuncture can have synergistic and additive benefits because both methods can affect the meridians, or energy channels, as well as the organs, systems, and elements of the body. Depending on the type, method, and length of cupping therapy and acupuncture—such as wet, dry, fire, moving, or stationary cupping—as well as the quantity, placement, manipulation, and depth of the needles—the integration of the two therapies can also have varying effects.

According to certain research, cupping therapy combined with acupuncture can be beneficial for a number of illnesses and ailments, including high blood pressure, osteoarthritis in the knee, chronic neck and low back pain, herpes zoster, and more. To evaluate the effectiveness and safety of cupping therapy plus acupuncture with other interventions, including acupuncture alone, cupping therapy alone, or a placebo, more research is necessary.

Massage

A massage is a manual therapy technique used to enhance blood circulation, reduce muscle tension, and calm the body and mind. It involves applying pressure, movement, and vibration to the body's soft tissues, including the muscles, tendons, ligaments, and fascia. By applying the cups to the same or adjacent areas as the massage, or by moving the cups along the meridians or the body's areas, cupping therapy can be combined with massage therapy to improve blood circulation, ease tension in the muscles, calm the body and mind, and treat or prevent a variety of illnesses and conditions, including pain, stress, fatigue, and more.

According to the laws of anatomy and physiology, the combination of cupping therapy and massage can have synergistic and advantageous benefits because both methods

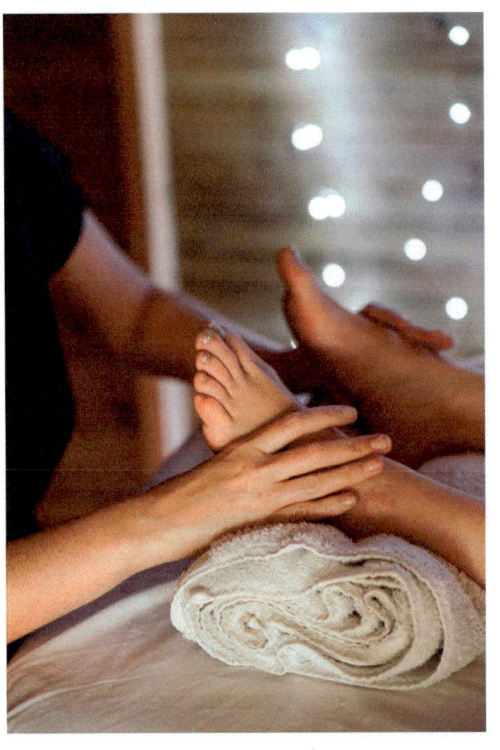

can affect the body's lymphatic drainage, muscular tone, blood flow, and neurological system. Depending on the type, method, and length of cupping therapy and massage— such as wet, dry, fire, moving, or stationary cupping—as well as the force, direction, and speed of the massage strokes, the integration of these two therapies

can also have varying effects.

According to certain research, cupping therapy combined with massage therapy can be beneficial for a number of illnesses and ailments, including cellulite, fibromyalgia, low back pain, shoulder discomfort, and chronic neck pain. To evaluate the effectiveness and safety of cupping therapy with massage with other interventions, including massage alone, cupping therapy alone, or a placebo, more research is necessary.

The Studies And Proof Of Cupping Therapy Using Innovative New Methods

Research on the use of novel techniques in cupping therapy, such as randomized controlled trials and meta-analyses, is another emerging trend in the field. By providing more credible and dependable evidence and results of cupping therapy and by addressing the shortcomings and gaps in the new research and evidence of cupping therapy, the research and evidence of cupping therapy using new methods can strengthen and validate the scientific and clinical basis and outcomes of cupping therapy. Researchers and practitioners may face new opportunities and challenges as a result of the research and evidence of cupping therapy using new methods. They can conduct and apply the research and evidence of cupping therapy, and they may also profit or lose out from it.

From a scientific and practical standpoint, there is some evidence, as well as instances of the research's advantages and disadvantages, and proof of cupping therapy using novel techniques. To compare cupping therapy with alternative interventions, like traditional cupping therapy, or no intervention at all, and to evaluate the quality and impact of the research and evidence of cupping therapy using modern methodologies, additional research and evidence are still required. Several techniques are available for investigating and substantiating cupping therapy, such as:

Randomized controlled trials

The goal of randomized controlled trials is to compare the benefits and effects of cupping therapy on a range of outcomes, including pain, inflammation, infection, and so on. Participants are randomized to either the intervention group, which receives cupping therapy, or the control group, which receives conventional therapies, sham cupping, or no intervention at all. Because randomized controlled trials account for confounding and biasing factors like the placebo effect, the expectation effect, or selection bias, they can strengthen and validate the scientific and clinical basis and outcomes of cupping therapy. They also provide more objective and rigorous evidence about the benefits of cupping therapy. Randomized controlled trials have several advantages, including:

- By evaluating the cupping therapy's mechanism and hypothesis, as well as by comparing the results and variations between the intervention and control groups, they can aid in proving the therapy's efficacy and causality. Statistical techniques like the p-value, confidence interval, and effect size can be used to measure and compare these variables.

- By randomly assigning participants and factors, like age, gender, or condition, as well as the kind, mode, and length of cupping therapy, to the intervention and control groups, and using randomization techniques like simple, stratified, or block randomization, they can help to lessen the unpredictability and uncertainty of cupping therapy.

- By following and abiding by the standards and guidelines—such as the CONSORT statement, the Cochrane handbook, or the PRISMA checklist—for the design, conduct, and reporting of randomized controlled trials, as well as by registering and publishing the protocols and the results of these trials in trial registries and peer-reviewed journals, they can contribute to increasing the validity and reliability of cupping therapy.

Some of the limitations of randomized controlled trials are:

- Conducting and implementing randomized controlled trials can be expensive and complex due to the need for additional resources and expertise, including time, money, and personnel, as well as equipment, software, and training. Additionally, there are ethical and practical issues to consider, such as participant recruitment, consent, and retention, as well as participant compliance, adherence, and dropout rates.

- More limitations and assumptions, such as inclusion and exclusion criteria, intervention and control conditions, or outcome measures, that might not accurately reflect real-world and clinical settings and scenarios, as well as greater heterogeneity and variability, such as participant characteristics, preferences, or responses, and the caliber, applicability, or relevance of the studies, that might compromise the external validity and applicability of randomized controlled trials, can make them hard to generalize and translate.

- More sources and forms of bias and error, such as allocation, performance, detection, or reporting bias, as well as random, systematic, or human error, can make them biased and difficult to interpret and evaluate. Moreover, more conflicts and controversies, like those involving study funding, sponsorship, or authorship, as well as the interpretation, dissemination, or application of the findings, can undermine the validity and usefulness of randomized controlled trials.

Meta-analyses:

In a meta-analysis, the data and findings from several studies—such as randomized controlled trials—that have examined the same or related questions or hypotheses—such as the efficacy and safety of cupping therapy for chronic neck pain—are gathered and analyzed. The results are then combined and summarized using statistical techniques like the mean difference, the standardized mean difference, or the odds ratio. Increasing the sample size, power, and generalizability of the studies, as well as giving more thorough and trustworthy data and results of cupping therapy, meta-analyses can strengthen and confirm the scientific and clinical basis and outcomes of the practice.

Among the advantages of meta-analyses are:

- Through systematic and transparent methods such as the search strategy, the inclusion and exclusion criteria, or the data extraction form, they can assist in synthesizing and integrating the evidence and outcomes of cupping therapy. They can do this by finding and identifying relevant and eligible studies (such as randomized controlled trials) that have looked into the same or similar questions or hypotheses.

- By using statistical techniques like the mean difference, the standardized mean difference, or the odds ratio to analyze and calculate the overall and subgroup effects and differences of cupping therapy on various outcomes, like pain, inflammation, infection, etc., they can aid in the quantification and comparison of the benefits and effects of the treatment. Additionally, they can evaluate and present the heterogeneity and variability of the effects and differences of cupping therapy using techniques like the I-squared, the Q-test, or the forest plot.

- By assessing the quality and risk of bias of the studies, such as the randomized controlled trials, that have looked into the benefits and effects of cupping therapy, they can help to assess and improve the quality and impact of the treatment. They can do this by using quality assessment tools, such as the Cochrane risk of bias tool, the GRADE approach, or the AMSTAR tool, and by identifying and addressing the gaps and limitations of the evidence and results of cupping therapy, such as by using sensitivity analysis, publication bias analysis, or meta-regression.

Among the drawbacks of meta-analyses are:

- The process of conducting and applying meta-analyses can be expensive and complex due to the need for additional resources and expertise, including personnel, money, and time, as well as equipment, software, and training. Additionally, there are additional ethical and practical considerations to consider, such as the availability, accessibility, and compatibility of study data and results, as well as the duplication, updating, or replication of meta-analyses.

- More restrictions and assumptions, such as inclusion and exclusion criteria, intervention and control conditions, or outcome measures, that might not accurately reflect real-world and clinical settings and scenarios, as well as more heterogeneity and variability, such as participant characteristics, preferences, or responses, and the caliber, applicability, or relevance of the studies, can make them hard to generalize and translate. These factors can also have an impact on the external validity and applicability of meta-analyses.

- More sources and forms of bias and error, such as selection, publication, or reporting bias, as well as random, systematic, or human error, can make meta-analyses more prone to bias and make them more difficult to interpret and evaluate. Moreover, more conflicts and controversies, such as those involving study funding, sponsorship, or authorship, as well as the interpretation, distribution, or application of the findings, can undermine the validity and usefulness of meta-analyses.

New status and trends of the regulation and standardization of Hijama cupping therapy

The degree of growth and acceptability of cupping therapy, along with legal, cultural, and social considerations, all influence how broadly and significantly cupping therapy is regulated and standardized in various nations, regions, and institutions. These are a few recent developments and trends regarding the standardization and regulation of cupping therapy:

- A number of well-established and comprehensive laws, rules, and policies that regulate and oversee the practice and research of cupping therapy, as well as more formal and standardized criteria, methods, and tools that assess the safety and quality of the treatment, are in place in some countries and regions, such as China, Egypt, the Middle East, and Africa, where cupping therapy is widely practiced and accepted. For instance, the Ministry of Health, the State Administration of Traditional Chinese Medicine, and the China Association of Acupuncture and Moxibustion, for instance, have issued and put into effect a number of rules, standards, and guidelines regarding the licensing, registration, and supervision of cupping practitioners, the categorization, manufacturing, and registration of cupping devices, and the planning, execution, and documentation of cupping research.

- Few comprehensive laws, rules, and policies that oversee and monitor the practice and research of cupping therapy, as well as informal and non-standardized criteria, methods, and tools that assess the safety and quality of the treatment, are in place in certain countries and regions, such as Europe, North America, and Australia, where cupping therapy is still relatively new, emerging, and less practiced and accepted. The regulation, standards, and guidelines for the qualification, certification, and supervision of cupping practitioners, the classification, specification, and registration of cupping devices, and the design, conduct, and reporting of cupping research vary widely across national and regional authorities, professional associations, and academic institutions in Europe, for instance.

- There are few or no laws, regulations, and policies that regulate and oversee the practice and research of cupping therapy, as well as few or nonexistent standards, procedures, and instruments that assess the safety and quality of the practice in some nations and regions, like India, Southeast Asia, and Latin America, where cupping therapy is comparatively unknown, unexplored, and rarely practiced and accepted. For instance, there are very few, if any, rules governing the training, certification, and supervision of cupping practitioners; the categorization, description, and registration of cupping devices; or the planning, execution, and documentation of cupping research in India. Moreover, there is no official or recognized authority or organization that regulates or standard sows cupping therapy practice.

The issues and risks associated with the absence or inadequacy of regulation and standardization of cupping Therapy

The need or insufficiency of the control and standardization of measuring treatment can pose different issues and dangers for the quality and security of measuring treatment, and the negligence or offense of measuring treatment. A few of the issues and dangers of the need or insufficiency of the control and standardization of measuring treatment are as follows:

- They can compromise and imperil the quality and security of measuring treatment, by permitting and empowering the utilization of substandard or imperfect measuring gadgets, such as cups, pumps, or valves, which will cause harm or damage to the patients, such as spillage, contamination, or burns of the cups, and by allowing and enduring the hone of unfit or inept measuring specialists, who may perform measuring treatment disgracefully or improperly, such as applying the glasses to the off-base or contraindicated ranges, or utilizing the off-base or intemperate weight or length of the cups.

- They can encourage and energize the negligence or offense of measuring treatment, by making and exploiting the escape clauses or crevices within the laws, rules, and approaches, that administer and screen the hone and inquire about measuring treatment, and by missing or disregarding the responsibility or obligation of the measuring specialists, who may mishandle or abuse measuring treatment for their claim advantage or intrigued, such as charging over the top or outlandish expenses, making untrue or overstated claims, or abusing the protection or privacy of the patients.

- They can weaken and ruin the validity and authenticity of measuring treatment, by falling flat or denying to supply or take after the benchmarks and rules, that degree and assess the quality and security of measuring treatment, and by missing or dismissing the proof and coming about, that bolster and validate the viability and benefits of measuring treatment, and by confronting or causing the feedback or resistance, from the open, the media, or the specialists, who may address or challenge the legitimacy and unwavering quality of measuring treatment.

The creation and enhancement of laws, regulations, and guidelines that oversee and keep an eye on the study and application of cupping therapy

The development and enhancement of laws, regulations, and policies that oversee and regulate the practice and research of cupping therapy can aid in addressing and mitigating the risks associated with the absence or insufficiency of cupping therapy regulation and standardization, as well as ensuring and enhancing the treatment's quality and safety and safeguarding and advancing the industry's rights and interests. The following are some examples of how laws, regulations, and policies that control and oversee the study and application of cupping therapy have been developed and improved:

- By developing and implementing laws, rules, and policies that regulate and standardize the training, certification, and supervision of cupping practitioners; the classification, specification, and registration of cupping devices; and the design, conduct, and reporting of cupping research, they can contribute to the establishment and maintenance of the safety and quality of cupping therapy. Additionally, they can enforce and inspect compliance with the laws, rules, and policies by the cupping practitioners, cupping devices, and cupping research; and they can impose and apply sanctions and penalties for breaking the laws, rules, and policies.

- Through the creation and implementation of laws, regulations, and policies that define and forbid the malpractice or misconduct of cupping therapy, such as fraud, deception, or negligence, as well as the establishment and management of mechanisms and procedures that identify and report such malpractice or misconduct—such as complaints, investigations, or lawsuits—as well as by providing and offering remedies and solutions—like compensation, restitution, or an apology—they can contribute to the prevention and reduction of cupping therapy-related malpractice and misconduct.

- They can contribute to strengthening and validating the legitimacy and credibility of cupping therapy by creating and enforcing laws, regulations, and policies that acknowledge and support the practice and research of cupping therapy as a legitimate and trustworthy form of complementary and alternative medicine. They can also collaborate and cooperate with other parties involved in the practice and research of cupping therapy, such as practitioners, researchers, patients, or authorities, and by raising and spreading public awareness of cupping therapy and its research.

Chapter 09

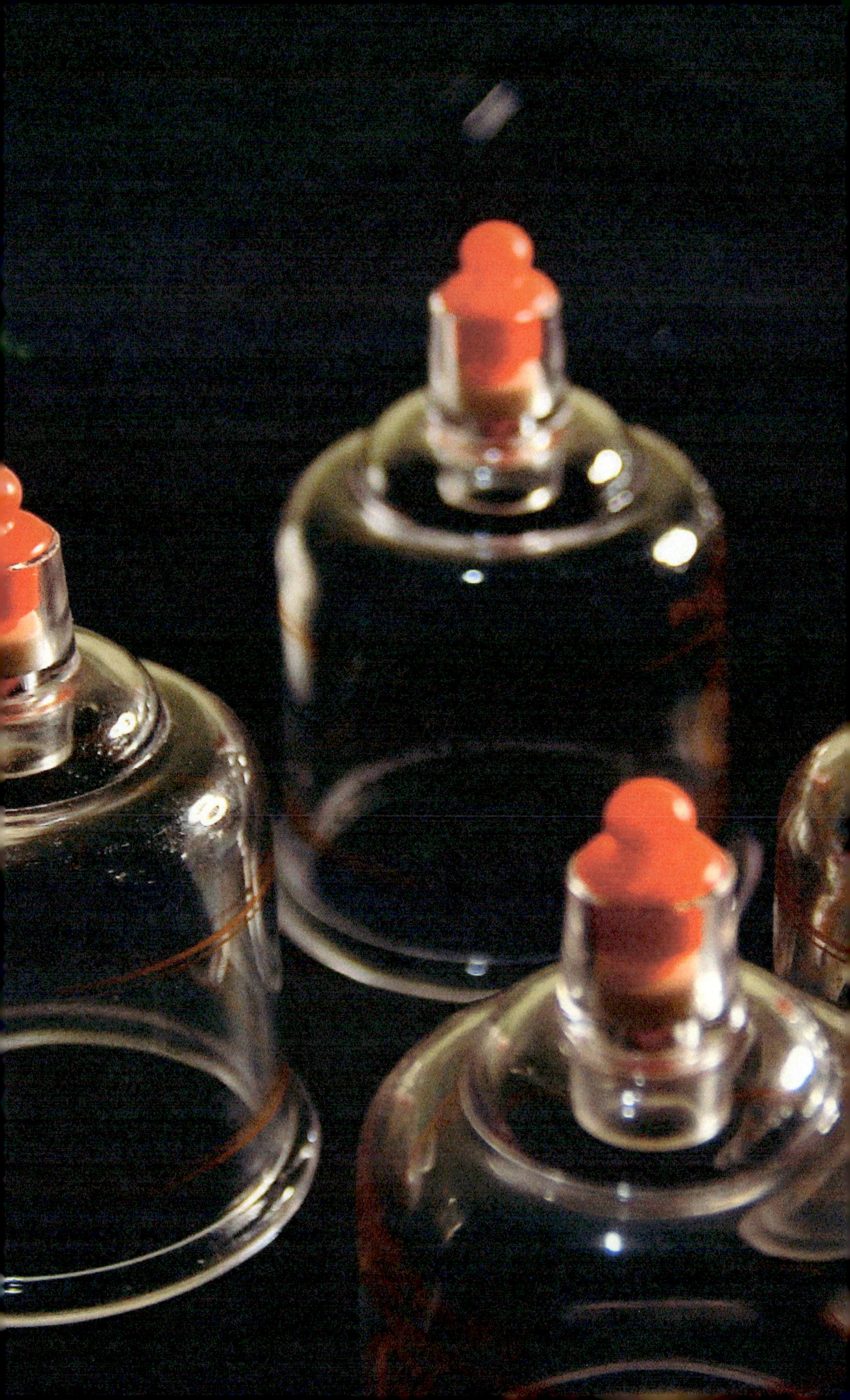

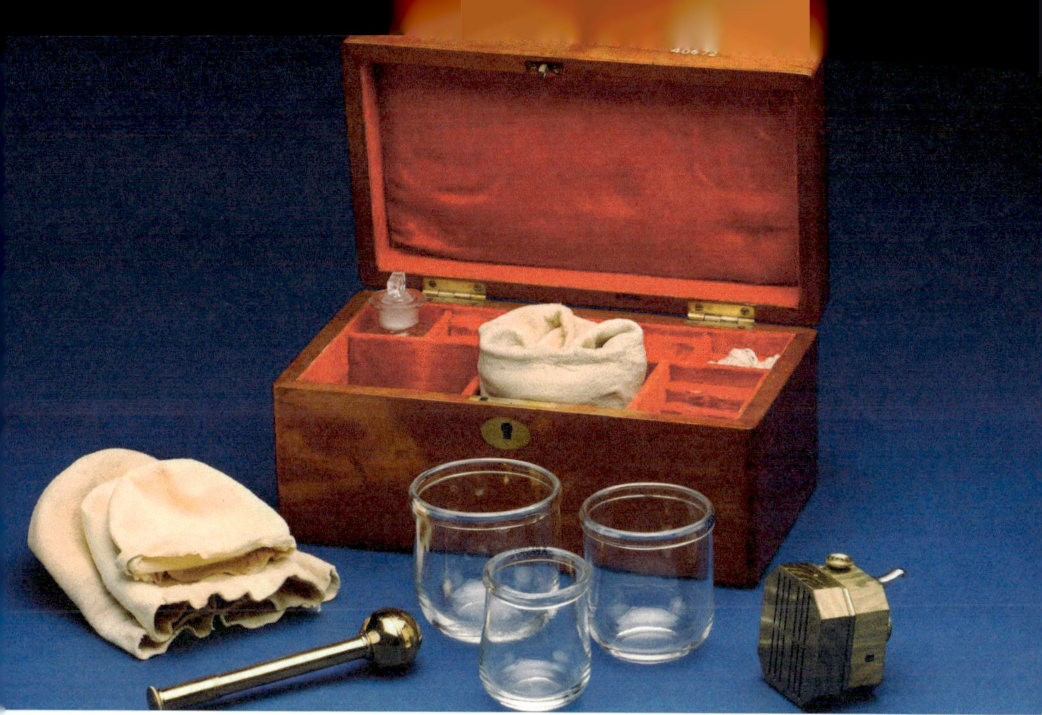

Myths and Misconceptions in Hijama Cupping Therapy

Which Hijama Cupping Therapy Myths, Misconceptions, and Cultural Variations Exist?

For thousands of years, Hijama cupping therapy has been used to treat or prevent a wide range of illnesses and ailments, including pain, inflammation, infection, skin issues, respiratory issues, digestive issues, and more, in a variety of cultures and geographical areas, including China, Egypt, the Middle East, Europe, and Africa.

Hijama cupping therapy is not without its myths and misunderstandings, though, as well as cultural variances.

These include erroneous or incorrect views or opinions, as well as various or varied customs or practices, all of which can have an impact on how Hijama cupping therapy is understood and used. Myths, misunderstandings, and cultural differences around Hijama cupping treatment are significant and pertinent because they can affect how Hijama cupping therapy is viewed and accepted as well as its efficacy and safety.

This chapter will cover common misunderstandings, myths, and cultural differences around Hijama cupping therapy, as well as how these things may impact knowledge and use of the technique. Along with learning to recognize and dispel myths and misconceptions, you will also gain an appreciation for and respect for the cultural differences in Hijama cupping therapy.

The myths and misconceptions in Hijama cupping therapy:

The myths and misunderstandings surrounding Hijama cupping therapy, or misleading or incorrect views or opinions that might mislead or confuse the public and experts regarding the nature and advantages of Hijama cupping therapy, present both opportunities and obstacles. Hijama cupping therapy myths and misunderstandings can be detrimental or beneficial, depending on how they are used or handled.

Some myths and misconceptions about Hijama cupping therapy are based on incomplete or distorted information or evidence, such as the practice's theory, history, or research; other myths and misconceptions are based on anecdotes, testimonials, or opinions about the practice that are based on the individual's subjective experience or preference.

The following are some widespread and popular myths and misconceptions regarding Hijama cupping therapy:

Hijama cupping treatment is either a superstition or a pseudoscience:

The idea that Hijama cupping therapy is a pseudoscience or superstition with no proof or scientific foundation, and that it depends on faith or magic to work, is a common misperception. This myth or misunderstanding may cause Hijama cupping therapy to be rejected or mocked, as well as cause people to be unaware of or deny its benefits.

This myth or misunderstanding is untrue or incorrect since Hijama cupping therapy is supported by evidence from science and reason rather than faith or magic to generate its desired results. The following are some examples of the rationale, scientific, or empirical support for Hijama cupping therapy:

- The practice of Hijama cupping therapy has a long history and is rooted in religious and cultural texts and practices such as the Quran, the Sunnah, the Bible, the Torah, and Ayurveda. It can be traced back to ancient times and civilizations such as China, Egypt, the Middle East, Europe, and Africa.

- Hijama cupping therapy has a sound theory and mechanism that is supported by ideas from modern medicine, such as the immune system, nervous system, and endocrine system, and that can be explained by traditional and alternative medicine concepts like energy balance, toxin removal, and blood flow stimulation.

- Research and evidence supporting the safety and efficacy of Hijama cupping therapy for a range of illnesses and conditions, including pain, inflammation, infection, and more, can be found through methods of scientific and clinical inquiry, such as case reports, meta-analyses, and randomized controlled trials.

Is Hijama cupping therapy a miracle treatment?

The idea that Hijama cupping therapy is a magic bullet, a panacea, capable of curing or preventing any illness, and superior to other forms of therapy or treatment is a common myth. This myth or fallacy may cause Hijama cupping therapy to be overused or misused, as well as to be neglected or without consideration for its restrictions and contraindications.

This is a myth or notion that is untrue or incorrect since Hijama cupping therapy is not a magic bullet that can treat or prevent any illness or condition or outperform any other form of therapy. A complementary or integrative therapy, Hijama cupping therapy can be used in conjunction with other therapies or modalities to augment or improve their benefits. The indications and contraindications of Hijama cupping therapy can help establish its appropriateness and usefulness for a variety of illnesses and ailments, as well as for various people and circumstances.

The following are some Hijama cupping therapy indications and contraindications:

- There are certain indications for the usage and efficacy of Hijama cupping therapy for a number of illnesses and ailments, including pain, inflammation, infection, skin issues, respiratory issues, digestive issues, and more. By boosting blood flow, eliminating toxins, and regulating energy levels in the body, Hijama cupping treatment can help improve or restore the functions and activities, as well as alleviate or lessen the symptoms and indications associated with certain diseases and ailments.

- Contraindications for Hijama cupping therapy include bleeding disorders, blood illnesses, heart disease, renal disease, pregnancy, and other circumstances for which it may not be suitable or acceptable. Hijama cupping therapy can result in blood loss, infection, or injury; it can also affect blood pressure, blood sugar, or blood clotting in the body. These factors can all contribute to or exacerbate the complications and side effects of these diseases and conditions, as well as interfere with their treatments and medications.

Hijama cupping therapy is a simple treatment?

The false belief is that Hijama cupping therapy is a simple technique that anyone can use at anytime, anywhere, and without the need for special training, knowledge, or abilities. This fallacy or misunderstanding raises the possibility of Hijama cupping therapy errors or misbehavior as well as the danger of complications and negative side effects.

This myth or fallacy is untrue or incorrect as Hijama cupping therapy is not a quick fix that can be used by anybody, anywhere, at any time, and without any special training, experience, or abilities. Hijama cupping therapy is a sophisticated and sensitive procedure that calls for expertise, training, and understanding to carry out correctly, safely, and with the least amount of difficulties and adverse effects possible. Hijama cupping treatment uses cups applied to the skin to create a vacuum inside the skin, which helps to balance the body's energy, eliminate toxins, and promote blood flow. To further cleanse and purify the body, Hijama cupping therapy also includes skin incisions and blood extractions.

The following are some of the abilities, know-how, and education needed for Hijama cupping therapy:

- **Skill:** Hijama cupping therapy requires skill in order to apply the cups to the right places on the body, create and modify the right pressure and duration for the cups, and incise and extract blood in a safe, hygienic manner using the right, sterile tools and techniques.

- **Knowledge:** Hijama cupping therapy requires knowledge in order to understand its theory and mechanism, as well as its effects and benefits on the body and mind. It also needs knowledge in order to identify the indications and contraindications, as well as its suitability and appropriateness for a variety of patients and situations, diseases, and conditions. Finally, knowledge is needed to manage any complications or side effects that may arise from Hijama cupping therapy as well as to prevent and treat them.

- **Training:** To learn and apply the principles, procedures, standards, and guidelines of Hijama cupping therapy, as well as its regulation and standardization, one must undergo training. Additionally, one must obtain and maintain current certification and qualification in Hijama cupping therapy, as well as seek out and receive supervision, feedback, and evaluation of the practice in order to improve it.

The differences in Hijama cupping therapy between cultures

The cultural variances in Hijama cupping therapy, or the many and varied customs or practices, are another facet and dimension of the therapy that can either reflect or impact its diversity and richness. Cultural differences in Hijama cupping treatment are significant and pertinent because they highlight the modality and integration of Hijama cupping therapy in various settings and cultures, as well as its distinctiveness and universality.

Hijama cupping therapy shows a number of cultural variations that can be seen and appreciated in the practice's various facets and tiers, including its historical and geographical origins and developments, its theoretical and philosophical underpinnings and frameworks, and its practical and clinical applications. Different factors and forces, such as religious and spiritual beliefs and values, social and political conditions and changes, and scientific and technological advancements and innovations, can also influence and affect these cultural variations.

The geographical, historical, and evolutionary roots of Hijama cupping therapy

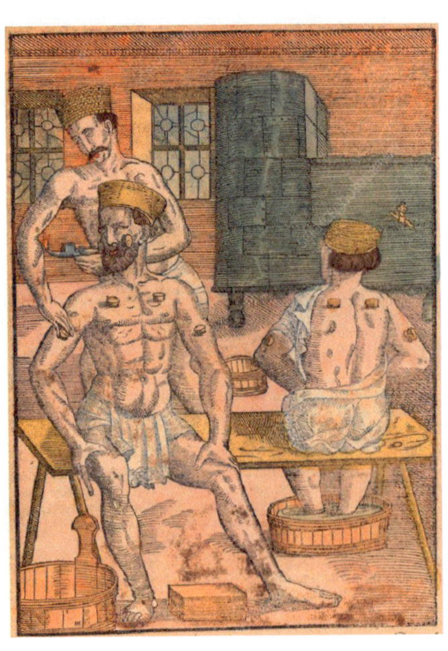

One of the cultural variations in Hijama cupping therapy is its historical and geographical origins and developments, which can be traced back to various civilizations, regions, and eras, including ancient Egypt, China, Greece, Rome, Persia, India, and so on. These origins and developments can also demonstrate how Hijama cupping therapy has evolved and adapted over time and space, including the introduction and spread of the practice by the Islamic prophet Muhammad and its innovation through integration with other modalities and technologies.

The historical and geographic origins and developments of

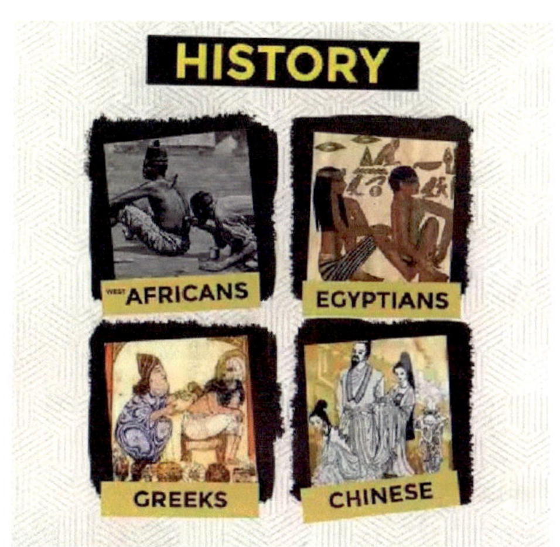

Hijama cupping therapy can reflect or have an impact on the diversity and richness of Hijama cupping therapy. They can reveal the similarities and differences, the influences and interactions, the opportunities and challenges, and the origins and history, transmission and diffusion, variation, and modification of Hijama cupping therapy in various cultures and contexts.

The following are some instances and supporting data on the historical and geographic roots and progressions of Hijama cupping therapy:

- The history and origins of Hijama cupping therapy can be found in ancient Egypt, China, Greece, Rome, Persia, India, and other ancient civilizations. These places are where Hijama cupping therapy was first used as a traditional and alternative medicine to treat and prevent a wide range of illnesses and conditions, including pain, inflammation, infections, and more. The Ebers Papyrus, the Huangdi Neijing, the Hippocratic Corpus, the De Medicina, the Canon of Medicine, the Sushruta Samhita, and other ancient texts and artifacts are a few examples of ancient books and artifacts that discuss or illustrate Hijama cupping therapy.

- The introduction and dissemination of Hijama cupping therapy can be traced back to the Islamic prophet Muhammad. He advocated and used Hijama cupping therapy as a prophetic and Islamic medical practice to treat and prevent a variety of illnesses and ailments, including fever, headaches, poisoning, and so forth. Several religious and cultural books and traditions, such as the Quran, the Sunnah, the Hadith, the Fiqh, etc., discuss or recommend Hijama cupping therapy.

- The ways in which Hijama cupping therapy has been modified and evolved include its incorporation and innovation with other modalities and technologies, including acupuncture, moxibustion, massage, herbal medicine, etc., to augment or enhance the effects and advantages of Hijama cupping therapy; additionally, it has been used to adapt or enhance its methods and techniques, such as the use of various cup types (glass, metal, bamboo, plastic, etc.); the use of various suction, fire, pump, and so on; and the use of various incisions (scalpel, lancet, blade, etc.).

The theoretical and philosophical frameworks and foundations of Hijama suction therapy

An additional aspect of cultural diversity observed in Hijama cupping therapy pertains to its philosophical and theoretical underpinnings and frameworks. These elements are distinct and varied, drawing from various medical systems, schools of thought, and knowledge sources. For instance, the Islamic medicine theory, the humoral theory, traditional Chinese medicine, Ayurvedic medicine, and traditional Chinese medicine theories are all present in Hijama cupping therapy.

The philosophical and theoretical underpinnings and frameworks of Hijama cupping therapy can either mirror or impact its diversity and abundance by demonstrating the various approaches and perspectives, explanations and interpretations, evidence and validations, and similarities and differences, influences and interactions, and challenges associated with Hijama cupping therapy across cultures and contexts.

The following are examples and evidence supporting the philosophical and theoretical frameworks and foundations of Hijama suction therapy:

- Based on ancient Greek and Roman medicine and philosophy, the humoral theory of Hijama cupping therapy posits that the human body is comprised of four humors—blood, phlegm, yellow bile, and black bile—and that the state of health or illness in the body is determined by the equilibrium or dysregulation of these humors. Through the incisions on the skin, Hijama cupping therapy can assist in balancing the humors by expelling detrimental or surplus humors, such as blood, from the body.

- The theory of Hijama cupping therapy, which is grounded in traditional Chinese medicine and ancient Chinese philosophy, posits that the human body is controlled by qi, or vital energy, which circulates through meridians or channels. Moreover, it asserts that the state of health or illness in the body is determined by the degree of harmony or discordance between qi and blood. Using the suction of the cups on the skin to stimulate the acupoints or points that correspond to the organs or functions on the meridians, Hijama cupping therapy can assist in balancing the qi and circulation.

- The ayurvedic cupping therapy theory, which is grounded in ancient Indian philosophy and medicine, posits that the human body is comprised of five panchamahabhutas (elementary states): earth, water, fire, air, and ether. The state of health or illness within the body is determined by the balance or imbalance of the three doshas (energys): vata, pitta, and kapha. Hijama cupping therapy can assist in the balancing of the doshas by expelling accumulated impurities or ama from the body via the skin incisions.

- The notion of Hijama cupping treatment in Islamic medicine is founded on the belief that Allah created the human body and that health and illness in the body are determined by compliance or noncompliance with Allah's directives and prohibitions. By following the prophet Muhammad's Sunnah, or the practice of the prophet, who performed and advocated for Hijama cupping therapy as a prophetic and Islamic medicine, and by using skin incisions to remove taiba, or harmful substances that affect the body and the soul, Hijama cupping therapy can aid in obeying Allah.

- Hijama cupping therapy is based on a modern medical theory that holds that the body is made up of cells, tissues, organs, and systems, and that the health and illness of the body are determined by how well or poorly these structures and functions work. Through the suction of the cups on the skin, Hijama cupping treatment can help to enhance function by activating the immunological and neurological systems, which control the body's defense and reaction, as well as by enhancing blood circulation and oxygenation, which feed and cure the body.

The therapeutic value and clinical implications of Hijama cupping Therapy

Another aspect of Hijama cupping therapy that varies depending on cultural preferences are the practical and clinical aspects and applications of the treatment. These can include the type, technique, and purpose of the Hijama cupping therapy, the decision, application, and frequency of the Hijama cupping therapy, the timing, location, and combination of the Hijama cupping therapy, the indications, contraindications, and precautions of the Hijama cupping therapy, the effects, benefits, and outcomes of Hijama cupping therapy, etc.

Hijama cupping therapy's practical and clinical aspects and applications can either reflect or have an impact on the therapy's diversity and richness by demonstrating the various options and choices, approaches and techniques, and outcomes and impacts of Hijama cupping therapy in various cultures and contexts, as well as by highlighting the parallels and divergences, influences and interactions, and opportunities and challenges of Hijama cupping therapy in various cultures and contexts. The following are some instances and supporting data about the clinical and practical uses and elements of Hijama cupping therapy:

- The goal and target, the condition and situation, the availability and accessibility of Hijama cupping therapy, as well as other considerations and preferences, can all influence the type, technique, and purpose of Hijama cupping therapy. Hijama cupping therapy comes in a variety of forms and techniques, including massage, dry, wet, flash, movement, and flash cupping. Each of these variations can be used for a variety of goals and outcomes, including stimulation, detoxification, and relaxation.

- Hijama cupping therapy selection, application, and frequency can vary based on a variety of criteria and preferences, including diagnosis and prescription, expertise and skill, and Hijama cupping therapy reaction and feedback. The number, size, and shape of the cups; the pressure, duration, and interval between the cups; the incision, extraction, and disposal of the blood; and other factors can all have an impact on the selection, application, and frequency of Hijama cupping therapy. These factors can also affect the efficacy, safety, and satisfaction of the practice.

- Several aspects and preferences, including the season and environment, the anatomy and physiology, and the compatibility and synergy of Hijama cupping therapy, can influence the timing, location, and combination of Hijama cupping therapy. The best and worst times and days, the most and least suitable points and areas, the most and least helpful modalities and therapies, etc., are just a few examples of recommendations and suggestions for the timing, location, and combination of Hijama cupping therapy. These recommendations and suggestions can have varying benefits and drawbacks, including the optimization, maximization, and minimization of Hijama cupping therapy.

- Hijama cupping therapy's indications, contraindications, and precautions might change based on a number of variables and preferences, including the patient's health and circumstances, the sickness and condition, and the potential risks and benefits of the procedure. The indications, contraindications, and precautions of Hijama cupping therapy are supported by a variety of evidences and examples. These include diseases and conditions like pain, inflammation, and infection that can be treated or prevented by Hijama cupping therapy; patients and situations that may be suitable or inappropriate for Hijama cupping therapy, including age, gender, pregnancy; and the risks and benefits that may be brought on by or avoided with Hijama cupping therapy, like bleeding, infection, injury, etc.

- Hijama cupping therapy can have a range of impacts, benefits, and outcomes based on a variety of characteristics and preferences, including assessment and evaluation, expectation and perception, and improvement and enhancement. Hijama cupping therapy effects, benefits, and outcomes can be measured and evaluated using a variety of criteria and techniques. These include subjective and objective, qualitative and quantitative, short- and long-term, and measures and indicators like blood pressure, quality of life, and pain scale that can demonstrate the effectiveness and value of Hijama cupping therapy.

Chapter 10

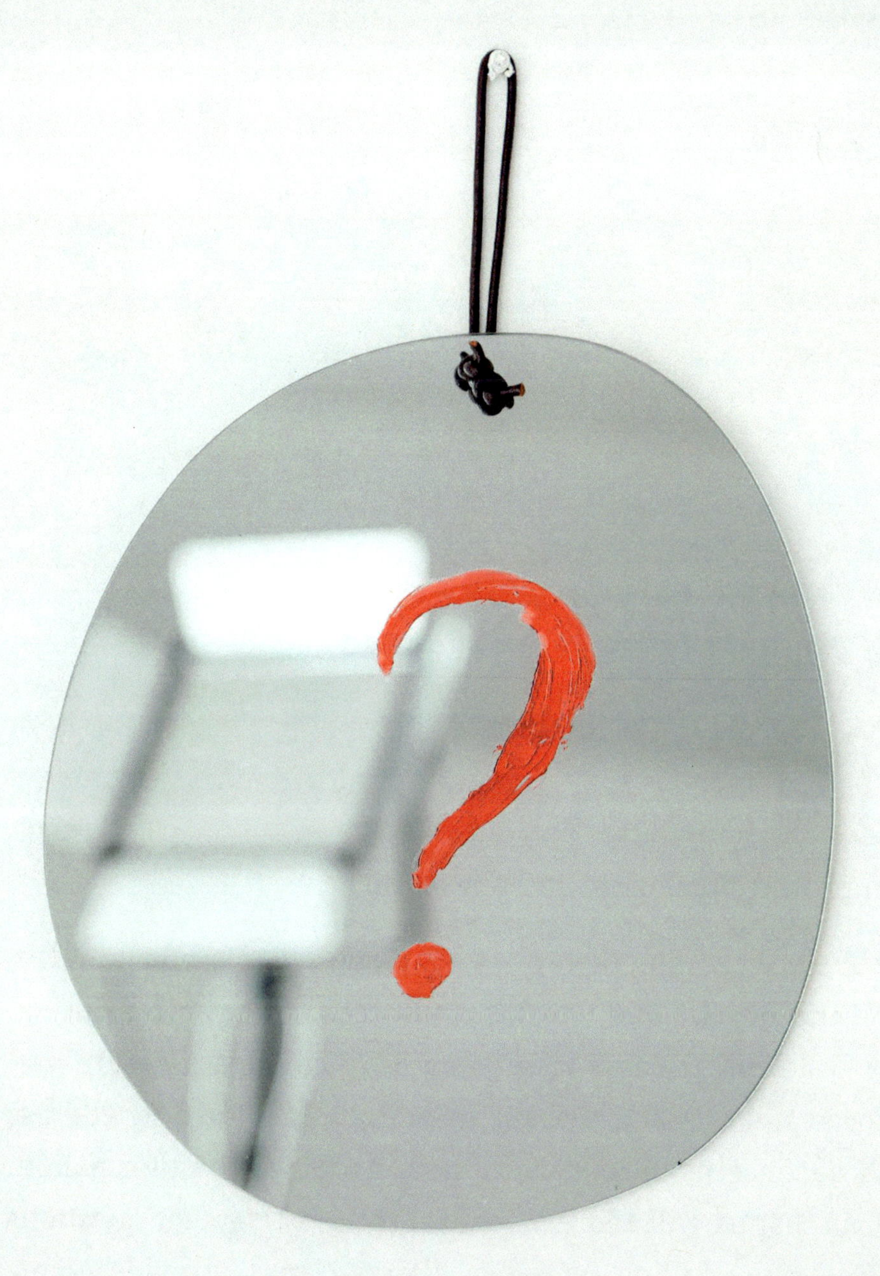

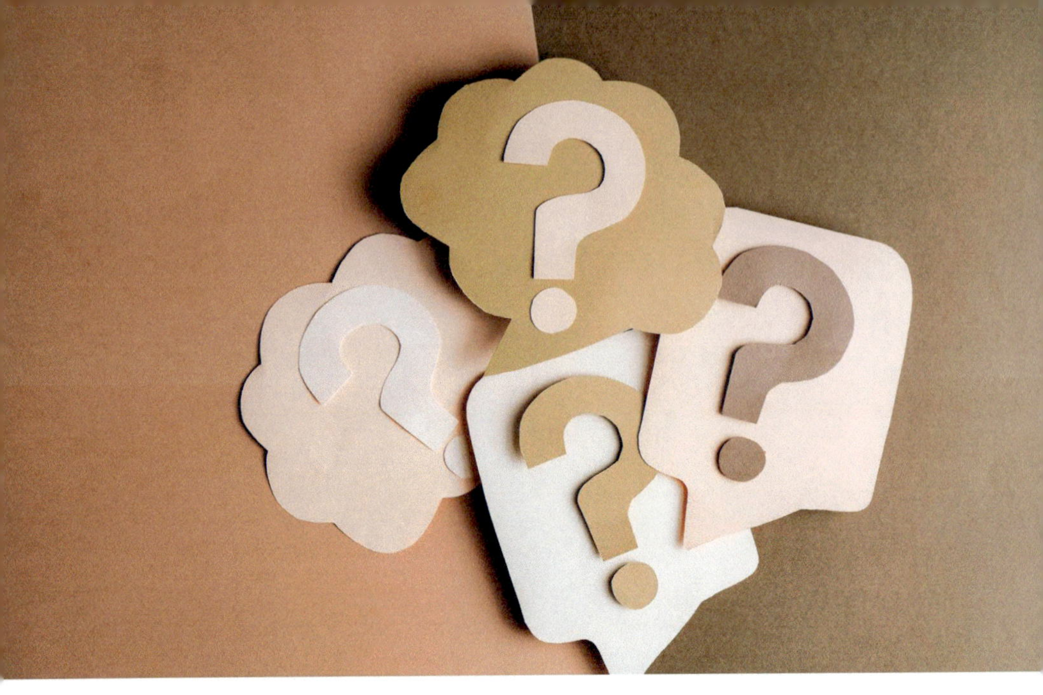

FAQs and Troubleshooting

Numerous advantages of cupping therapy for both mental and physical health include increased immunity, decreased inflammation, pain relief, improved circulation, and relaxation.

But since cupping therapy is not a one-size-fits-all approach, several queries and worries could come up prior to, during, or following a cupping session. To guarantee a secure and successful cupping therapy session, it is critical to address these concerns and offer accurate and trustworthy information. This chapter will address some of the most popular questions (FAQs) regarding cupping therapy and provide some troubleshooting advice for typical issues or difficulties.

Frequently Asked Questions (FAQs)

Q: How does cupping therapy combine with conventional medical treatments?

Ans: Cupping therapy is not a replacement for established medical treatments, but rather a complimentary therapy that can improve the effectiveness of traditional medicine. Cupping treatment can aid in the absorption and distribution of pharmaccuticals, lessen drug adverse effects, and promote the body's natural healing processes. Cupping therapy should not be used on areas with injections, implants, or surgical incisions since it might induce problems or infections. Cupping therapy should also be avoided for those who are on blood thinners, have bleeding problems, or have low blood pressure, since it may increase the risk of bleeding or bruising. It is best to contact with your doctor before starting cupping treatment, especially if you have any pre-existing medical issues or are taking any drugs.

Q: Can cupping treatment be tailored to specific medical conditions?

Ans: Yes, cupping therapy may be tailored to a specific health problem by changing the kind, quantity, size, and positioning of the cups, as well as the duration and strength of suction. Depending on the health situation, multiple cupping procedures may be required, such as dry cupping, wet cupping, movement cupping, and flash cupping. Dry cupping, for example, is appropriate for overall wellbeing and relaxation; wet cupping is great for detoxification and blood purification; moving cupping is beneficial for muscular tension and pain alleviation; and flash cupping is beneficial for respiratory problems and asthma. Furthermore, different health situations may necessitate distinct cupping spots, which are based on acupuncture and reflexology concepts. Cupping points on the back may stimulate the lungs, kidneys, liver, and spleen, whilst cupping points on the legs can stimulate the digestive, urinary, and reproductive systems. A competent and experienced cupping therapist can assist you in determining the most appropriate cupping method and sites for your particular health condition.

Q: Is cupping therapy appropriate for children, and are there any age-related concerns?

Ans: Cupping treatment is appropriate for children as long as they are old enough to comprehend and cooperate with the procedure, and they have parental permission and supervision. Cupping treatment can benefit children with a variety of health concerns, including colds, coughs, allergies, asthma, digestive disorders, skin ailments, and behavioral challenges. However, there are several age-related factors to consider while practicing cupping treatment on children. Children's skin is more fragile and sensitive than adults', thus the cups should be smaller, softer, and less pressured, with gentle and short suction. Second, because children's bodies are more active and energetic than adults', the cups should be put in regions where they are unlikely to move or be disturbed, and the session should be shorter and less frequent. Third, because children have stronger emotional and psychological reactions than adults, the cups should be introduced gradually and cautiously, with the therapist explaining the technique and its advantages in a straightforward and comforting manner, and monitoring the child's comfort and feedback during the session.

Q: What impact do food and nutrition have prior to and following cupping therapy?

Ans: Diet and nutrition are significant factors in preparing for and recovering from cupping therapy because they influence the quality and amount of blood and fluids brought to the skin's surface. Before receiving cupping therapy, it is advised that you eat a light and nutritious meal that includes fruits, vegetables, grains, and lean meats, as well as drink lots of water to hydrate and nourish your body. It is also recommended that you avoid meals that are spicy, fatty, fried, processed, or heavy in sugar, salt, or caffeine, since they might induce indigestion, inflammation, or discomfort. Following cupping therapy, it is recommended that you consume foods high in iron, vitamin C, and antioxidants, such as spinach, broccoli, citrus fruits, berries, and almonds, to replace and heal the blood and tissues. It is also advised that you drink extra water to flush out the toxins and waste materials produced by cupping treatment, and that you avoid alcohol, smoke, and narcotics, since these might interfere with the healing process or induce bad responses.

Q: Do cupping procedures vary according on cultural or regional practices?

Ans: Yes, cupping procedures vary depending on cultural or regional practices, as cupping treatment has been used for thousands of years and has been impacted by numerous traditions, beliefs, and customs. Some of the differences in cupping techniques are:

- The kind and shape of the cups: Depending on the client's and therapist's preferences, cupping treatment can employ cups that are round, oval, square, or triangular, as well as cups made of glass, metal, bamboo, ceramic, plastic, or silicone.

- The process of producing suction: Depending on the kind of cups and the required pressure, cupping therapy might use fire, pumps, valves, or rubber bulbs to produce suction.

- The position and quantity of the cups: Depending on the goal and extent of the treatment, cupping therapy might involve placing the cups on the back, neck, shoulders, arms, legs, belly, chest, or face. There can also be one to several dozen cups used.

- The length and frequency of the sessions: Depending on the ailment and therapeutic aim, cupping therapy sessions can range from a few minutes to an hour, and they can be done once or multiple times a week, month, or year.

- Combination with other therapies: To maximize the advantages and effects of treatment, cupping therapy can be coupled with other therapies like massage, acupuncture, herbal medicine, or aromatherapy.

Q: Can cupping therapy help with mental health disorders like stress and anxiety?

Ans: Cupping therapy can help with mental health disorders like stress and anxiety by increasing the release of endorphins, serotonin, and dopamine, which are natural chemicals that govern mood, emotion, and cognition. Cupping therapy can also stimulate the parasympathetic neural system, which is responsible for the relaxation response, while inhibiting the activity of the sympathetic nervous system, which is responsible for the stress reaction. Cupping therapy can assist to relax the mind, relieve stress, and regulate emotions, improving the individual's mental health and quality of life.

Q: How does cupping therapy impact the lymphatic system and circulation?

Ans: Cupping therapy stimulates the lymphatic system and circulation by boosting blood flow and lymphatic drainage in the area where the cups are placed. The suction induced by the cups dilates and expands the blood arteries and capillaries, allowing the blood and fluids to move more freely. This enhances the transport of oxygen and nutrients to cells and tissues while also removing carbon dioxide and waste from the body. Cupping therapy also activates the lymph nodes and glands, which are part of the immune system, allowing them to filter and remove toxins and pathogens that might cause infections or illnesses. Cupping therapy can thereby improve the health and function of the lymphatic system and circulation while also preventing or treating a variety of illnesses such as edema, cellulitis, varicose veins, hypertension, and arthritis.

Q: Are there any special precautions to take when receiving cupping therapy when pregnant?

Ans: Yes, pregnant people should take special precautions when seeking cupping therapy since pregnancy causes major changes in the body and hormones that may impact the treatment's reaction and result. Pregnant individuals should avoid cupping therapy during the first trimester due to the critical period for fetal development and the risk of complications or miscarriage.

- Cupping therapy should not be used on the belly, lower back, or sacrum since these regions are related with the uterus, ovaries, and fallopian tubes, and any pressure or manipulation might cause contractions or preterm delivery.

- Cupping therapy should not be used on the breasts since they are delicate and susceptible to engorgement, mastitis, and infection, and any suction or irritation may cause pain or injury to the nipples or milk ducts.

- Cupping therapy should be executed by a qualified and experienced cupping therapist who understands the anatomy and physiology of pregnancy and can adjust the type, number, size, and placement of the cups, as well as the duration and intensity of the suction, based on the pregnancy's stage and status.

Q: Can cupping therapy help manage chronic pain conditions?

Ans: Cupping therapy can help manage chronic pain illnesses including fibromyalgia, osteoarthritis, rheumatoid arthritis, sciatica, and migraines by lowering inflammation, increasing blood circulation, relaxing muscles, and releasing endorphins. Cupping therapy can help relieve the pain and stiffness associated with chronic pain problems while also improving joint and limb function. Cupping therapy can also aid to alter pain signal perception and transmission in the brain and spinal cord, as well as lessen the sensitivity and threshold of pain receptors throughout the body. Cupping therapy can thus serve as a natural and non-invasive alternative or supplement to traditional pain drugs, which may have adverse effects or dependence difficulties.

Q: What scientific evidence supports the effectiveness of cupping therapy?

Ans: Cupping therapy has been the topic of several scientific research investigations, both in vitro and in vivo, as well as in humans and animals, demonstrating its usefulness for a variety of health issues and results. Research suggests that cupping therapy can improve oxygen delivery and utilization by increasing hemoglobin, hematocrit, and red blood cell levels in the bloodstream. (Al Bedah et al., 2019)

- Cupping therapy can lower levels of inflammatory cytokines including interleukin-6 and tumor necrosis factor-alpha, which can regulate the immune response and inflammation in the body. (Farahmand et al, 2014)

- Cupping therapy can boost nitric oxide levels, which relaxes smooth muscles and dilates blood vessels, improving blood flow and pressure in the body. (Mamoud et al., 2015)

- Cupping therapy can boost levels of antioxidants like glutathione and superoxide dismutase, which protect cells and tissues from oxidative stress and damage. (El Sayed et al., 2017).

- Cupping therapy can lower cortisol levels, a stress hormone that affects the body's metabolism, immunity, and mood. (Michelsen et al., 2009)

- When compared to other therapies, cupping therapy can enhance the quality of life, pain severity, and functional status of individuals with persistent low back pain. (Kim et al. 2011)

Cupping therapy can enhance the clinical symptoms, lung function, and quality of life of individuals with chronic obstructive pulmonary disease when compared to traditional therapies. Cao et al., 2011.

- Cupping therapy can reduce the frequency, intensity, and duration of migraine attacks when compared to other therapies. (Ahangar et al., 2019.)

Q: How may seasoned cupping practitioners be distinguished from inexperienced ones?

Ans: The following characteristics can help distinguish between seasoned cupping practitioners and beginners:

- The cupping practitioner's credentials and certification: A skilled cupping practitioner should be able to produce documentation of their education and experience, as well as a legitimate and acknowledged qualification and certification in cupping therapy, such as from a respectable cupping association, organization, or institution.

- The practitioner of cupping's background and reputation: An expert cupping practitioner should be able to give references or testimonies from their past or present customers, as well as sufficient and pertinent experience in cupping therapy, as measured by the number of years, hours, or cases completed.

- The knowledge and expertise of the cupping practitioner: A skilled and knowledgeable cupping practitioner should possess thorough and current knowledge and expertise in cupping therapy, including the types, techniques, points, and indications of cupping. They should also be able to accurately and clearly explain the process and its advantages.

- The cupping practitioner's hygiene and reliability: A skilled cupping practitioner should adhere to the cupping therapy's hygiene and safety standards and guidelines, which include using sterile, disposable cups and equipment, donning gloves and masks, thoroughly cleaning and disinfecting the cupping area, and appropriately disposing of waste.

- The cupping practitioner's interaction and rapport: A skilled cupping practitioner should be able to listen to their clients' needs and expectations, address any questions or concerns they may have, get their permission and feedback, and respect their comfort and privacy.

Q: Is there a suggested cupping session frequency to achieve the best possible results?

Ans: Depending on the condition, aim, reaction, and preference of the individual, there is no set recommendation for the number of cupping sessions that will yield the best results. Nonetheless, the following broad principles might assist in deciding how frequently to hold cupping sessions:

- Cupping sessions can be performed once or twice a month, or as needed, to preserve the body and mind's equilibrium and overall well-being.

- Cupping sessions can be done once or twice a week, or until the symptoms go away, for mild to moderate acute diseases including colds, coughs, headaches, or muscular spasms. This can help to reduce discomfort and hasten healing.

- Cupping sessions can be done twice or three times a week, or until the disease improves, to reduce inflammation and discomfort and improve function and quality of life for severe or chronic disorders such diabetes, hypertension, asthma, arthritis, or asthma.

- Cupping sessions can be done once or twice a year, or more frequently as suggested by the cupping practitioner, to help detoxify and purify the body and mind.

Q: Can cupping therapy help athletes and sports-related injuries?

Ans: Yes, cupping therapy can benefit athletes and sports-related ailments by improving their physical and mental performance as well as recuperation. Cupping treatment improves athletes by increasing blood flow and oxygen supply to muscles and tissues, improving strength, endurance, and stamina.

Cupping therapy helps relieve muscular tension and pain, allowing athletes to enhance their flexibility, mobility, and coordination.

- Cupping treatment stimulates the release of endorphins, which improves athletes' mood, motivation, and confidence.

- Cupping therapy helps speed up the recovery of sports injuries including sprains, strains, bruises, and fractures by lowering inflammation, swelling, and discomfort while also stimulating cell and tissue regeneration.

- Cupping treatment can help to prevent or treat sports-related disorders including weariness, cramps, spasms, and dehydration by restoring body-mind balance.

Cupping therapy may thus be a useful and successful treatment for athletes and sports-related ailments, and many professional and amateur athletes have integrated it into their training and recuperation regimens.

Q: What measures should those who have skin issues take before cupping?

Ans: People with skin diseases like eczema, psoriasis, acne, or herpes should exercise caution before cupping since it may worsen or infect their skin disorders. Before cupping, persons with skin disorders should consult with their dermatologist and cupping practitioner to discuss their skin condition and medical history. Seek their advice and consent for cupping.

- Avoid cupping on current sores, wounds, or infections, since this might exacerbate the disease or transfer the infection to other places or persons.

- Choose a competent and experienced cupping practitioner who adheres to cupping's hygiene and safety standards and requirements, such as utilizing sterile and disposable cups and equipment, using gloves and masks, cleaning and sanitizing the cupping space, and appropriately disposing of waste.

- Apply a moisturizer or soothing lotion to the skin before and after cupping to keep it hydrated and protected from dryness or irritation.

- Monitor their skin's state and reaction to cupping, and report any signs of worsening or infection, such as redness, swelling, pus, or fever, to their dermatologist and cupping practitioner. Seek emergency medical assistance if necessary.

Q: Are there any cultural or religious concerns for cupping therapy?

Ans: Cupping treatment is a global and inclusive therapy that everyone may practice and enjoy, regardless of culture or religion. However, cupping treatment may have certain special cultural or religious implications, since it has been impacted by numerous traditions, beliefs, and rituals. Some of the special cultural or religious factors associated with cupping treatment include:

- The Origins and History of Cupping Therapy: Cupping treatment is said to have started in ancient China as a kind of acupuncture and herbal medicine, before spreading to other regions of Asia, Africa, Europe, and America, where it was accepted and adapted by many nations and civilizations. Cupping therapy, for example, was done by the ancient Egyptians, Greeks, and Romans, who utilized animal horns, shells, or earthenware as cups, as well as the Islamic prophet Muhammad, who supported cupping as a treatment for a variety of diseases and employed glass or metal cups.

- Cupping therapy terminology and symbolism: Cupping therapy can have many names and connotations in different languages and cultures, depending on its origin and history. Cupping treatment, for example, is known as hijama in Arabic, which means "sucking" and is regarded a sunnah, or a practice of the prophet Muhammad, as well as a form of devotion and healing in Islam. Cupping treatment, also known as ba guan in Chinese, which means "eight trigrams," is related with the notions of yin and yang, as well as the balance of energy and forces in the body and nature in Taoism.

- Cupping therapy etiquette and ethics: Cupping therapy rules and laws vary among countries and faiths, based on societal values and customs. Cupping therapy, for example, may require the consent and permission of the spouse, family, or community, particularly for women, children, or the elderly, and may respect the client's privacy and modesty, particularly in sensitive or sacred areas such as the head, face, chest, or genitals. Cupping therapy may also need the adherence of certain rituals or prayers, such as chanting God's name or the therapy's objective or purpose, prior to, during, or after the session.

Q: Can cupping therapy help with detoxification, and how does it work?

Ans: Yes, cupping treatment can help with detoxification, which is the process of eliminating or neutralizing toxins and waste products that build up in the body due to a variety of causes such as nutrition, lifestyle, environment, or illness. Cupping therapy can aid in detoxification by stimulating blood circulation and lymphatic drainage. This helps transport toxins and waste products from cells and tissues to detoxifying organs like the liver, kidneys, lungs, skin, and colon.

- Inducing micro-traumas and inflammations on the skin, which activates the immune system and the inflammatory response, allowing it to mobilize and eliminate toxins and pathogens that might cause infections or illnesses.

- Drawing the blood and fluids containing toxins and waste materials to the skin's surface, where they may be removed or absorbed by the cups, particularly in wet cupping, which punctures the skin and extracts the blood by suction.

Q. How does cupping therapy affect the immune system?

Ans: Cupping therapy affects the immune system, which is the body's natural defensive mechanism against external invaders including bacteria, viruses, fungus, and parasites that can cause illnesses or diseases. Cupping therapy boosts the immune system by increasing white blood cell production and activity, as well as antibodies that recognize and neutralize foreign invaders. This improves the body's immunity and resistance.

- Changing the balance and function of the immune system, which can be hyperactive or underactive, resulting in autoimmune illnesses like rheumatoid arthritis, lupus, or multiple sclerosis, as well as immunodeficiency disorders like AIDS or cancer. Cupping treatment can help control and normalize the immune system while also preventing or treating immunological-related disorders.

- Inducing the production of cytokines, which are chemical messengers that communicate and coordinate the immune system while also influencing inflammation, healing, and regeneration. Cupping therapy can help raise anti-inflammatory cytokines, which reduce inflammation and discomfort, while decreasing pro-inflammatory cytokines, which induce chronic inflammation and tissue damage.

Cupping therapy can therefore affect the immune system by strengthening and regulating it while also enhancing inflammation, healing, and regeneration in the body.

Q: What does cupping mean by the markings it leaves behind, and does it mean that the injury has healed?

Ans: The markings left by cupping are the result of the force and vacuum created by the cups, which push fluids and blood to the skin's surface, causing bubbles, lumps, and discolorations.

Although the markings produced by cupping have some significance, they are not always indicative of recovery. The following are some interpretations and implications of the markings made by cupping:

- Color and intensity of the markings: Depending on the amount and quality of blood and other fluids that are brought to the skin's surface, the color and intensity of the markings left by cupping can vary, ranging from pale pink to dark violet. In general, the more pollutants and waste products there are in the body, as well as the more congestion and restriction in the region where the cups are placed, the darker and stronger the markings. There are less pollutants and waste materials in the body and greater blood flow and movement in the area where the cups are placed if the markings are lighter and less intense.

- The shape and size of the markings: Depending on the kind and size of the cups, as well as the length and force of the suction, the shapes and sizes of the marks created by cupping can vary, ranging from round to elliptical and microscopic to enormous. In general, more damage and stress to the tissues and organs is indicated by larger and more unequal markings, which also indicate more edema and inflammation in the region where the cups are placed.

The length and regularity of the marks: Depending on the condition, response, and recovery of the individual, the length and regularity of the marks left by cupping can vary, ranging from a few hours to a few weeks, and from once to several times. The smaller and more even the marks, the less inflammation and edema that are in the area where the cups are applied, and the less harm and trauma that are in the tissues and organs.

In general, the more persistent and severe the problem being treated with cupping, the longer and more regular the markings, and the more difficult and delayed the healing process will be. The problem being treated by cupping is less severe and chronic the shorter and less regular the markings are, and the healing process is also more rapid and simple.

Q: Are there particular things that people with blood clotting issues need to be aware of?

Ans: Due to the increased risk of bleeding or bruises, those with blood coagulation problems, such as hemophilia, thrombophilia, or von Willebrand disease, should exercise extreme caution when undergoing cupping therapy. Some special concerns for people with blood clotting problems include: - Before cupping, discuss your blood clotting disorder and medical history with your hematologist and cupping practitioner. Ask for their advice and consent.

Steer clear of wet cupping, which entails making punctures in the skin to draw blood, since this might result in infection or excessive or prolonged bleeding. Blood clotting problems patients may find dry cupping, which does not need skin breaking, to be a safer option.

- Select a licensed and skilled cupping professional who complies with all safety and hygienic regulations. This includes utilizing sterile, disposable cups and equipment, using gloves and masks, thoroughly cleaning and sanitizing the cupping space, and appropriately disposing of waste.

- After the session, apply a pressure bandage or a cold compress to the cupping area to prevent or treat swelling or inflammation, as well as to stop or lessen bleeding or bruising.

- After cupping, keep an eye on the blood clotting status and response. Notify your hematologist and cupping practitioner of any unusual or severe bleeding or bruising, including hematomas, hematuria, hemoptysis, or hematemesis, and seek emergency medical assistance if needed.

Q: Is it possible to combine cupping therapy with other complementary therapies, like acupuncture?

Ans: It is possible to combine cupping therapy with other complementary therapies, such acupuncture. Acupuncture is an ancient therapeutic method that involves putting tiny needles into certain body locations to promote balance and energy in the body and mind. Given that both acupuncture and cupping therapy are based on reflexology and acupuncture principles and affect the flow and circulation of blood and energy in the body and mind, they can have beneficial and synergistic effects. Depending on the health and choice of the patient, as well as the aim and objective of the therapy, cupping therapy and acupuncture may be conducted on the same or separate sites. These are some potential synergies and factors to take into account when combining therapies. For example, cupping treatment and acupuncture can be used to the same sites to maximize their stimulation and impact, or to separate points to target other body and mind systems or areas.

- Depending on the kind and technique of cupping and acupuncture, as well as the client's and therapist's availability and expertise, cupping treatment and acupuncture may be administered sequentially or concurrently. For instance, cupping therapy and acupuncture can be administered simultaneously, like putting in the needles first and then applying the cups, or vice versa, to produce a deeper and stronger effect on the body and mind, or in the opposite order, such as cupping first and then acupuncture, or vice versa, to prepare or reinforce the body and mind for the therapy.

- Depending on the illness, reaction, and recovery of the individual, cupping therapy and acupuncture may have complimentary or opposing effects and consequences. Cupping therapy and acupuncture, for instance, can have contradictory or complementary effects, such as aggravating the condition or symptoms, causing overstimulation or exhaustion, causing bleeding or infection, or decreasing inflammation and pain while increasing blood flow and energy flow.

Q: How long do the effects of cupping therapy usually remain between sessions?

Ans: The advantages of cupping therapy usually endure between sessions, depending on the patient's condition, aim, reaction, and recuperation. However, there are certain broad recommendations that might assist predict the length of the advantages of cupping therapy.

- The advantages of cupping therapy for overall wellness and prevention might last from a few days to a few weeks, or until the next session, depending on the individual's health and lifestyle, as well as the frequency and intensity of the cupping sessions.

- Cupping therapy can provide advantages for acute or moderate ailments for a few hours to a few days, or until the problem resolves, depending on the severity and etiology of the condition, as well as the frequency and length of the cupping sessions.

- For chronic or severe disorders, the advantages of cupping therapy can continue from a few days to a few months, or until the condition improves, depending on the type and origin of the ailment, as well as the frequency and consistency of cupping sessions.

These are some broad recommendations for estimating the length of the advantages of cupping therapy, and one should always monitor and assess their health and development, adjusting their treatment plan as needed.

Troubleshooting Common Concerns:

Cupping therapy is a safe and effective therapy that can improve both physical and emotional health. However, cupping therapy might produce small or transient side effects or problems such as bruising, soreness, infection, or emotional responses. These difficulties are often not significant or damaging, and can be readily avoided or controlled with adequate care and communication. However, in certain rare or unique circumstances, cupping therapy may cause unusual or dangerous responses or complications, such as allergic reactions, medical crises, or legal challenges. These difficulties demand quick attention and expert action; they should not be overlooked or neglected. This section will give some troubleshooting advice and information for frequent and rare difficulties that may develop during cupping therapy sessions, and help you deal with them efficiently and securely.

A. Bruising and Marking:

- It is normal and anticipated for cupping therapy to result in bruises and markings because the pressure and suction of the cups push blood and fluids to the skin's surface, where they form welts, blisters, and discolorations.

- Depending on the person's health, reaction, and recuperation, bruises and markings often go away in a few days or weeks and are neither hazardous or dangerous.

- Although they may be significant and indicate something, bruises and marks do not always indicate recovery. The quantity and quality of the blood and fluids, the kind and technique of cupping, the position and quantity of cups, the person's health and lifestyle, and the marks themselves may all affect the color, intensity, form, size, duration, and frequency of the markings.

Here are some pointers to reduce or control bleeding and scarring:

- Before and after cupping, use a moisturizing or calming lotion to nourish and shield the skin from dryness or irritation.

- After the session, apply a pressure bandage or a cold compress to the cupping area to prevent or treat swelling or inflammation, as well as to stop or lessen bleeding or bruising.

- To nourish and replenish the blood and tissues, as well as to flush out the toxins and waste products generated by cupping, drink lots of water and eat a nutritious diet.

- Steer clear of the sun, heat, and cold since these factors might exacerbate skin discoloration or irritation.

- Steer clear of narcotics, alcohol, smoke, and extreme

physical activity since they might impede the healing process or have unfavorable effects.

- Several indications or symptoms that might point to a major issue or severe bruising include:

- The markings are painful, big, uneven, black, and persistent.

- They do not go away with time.

- Fever, rash, pus, infection, or the markings spread to other persons or places go along with the marks.

- Wet cupping is the cause of the markings, and the blood is extremely thick, black, or clotted, or it may contain contaminants or foreign objects.

- The patient has a history of medical issues, or they are on medication (blood thinners, thrombophilia, hemophilia) that affects blood clotting or circulation.

- Hematomas, hematuria, hemoptysis, or hematemesis are examples of abnormal or excessive bleeding or bruising in other areas of the body that the person experiences.

It is imperative that you cease cupping immediately and seek expert medical treatment as soon as possible if you encounter any of these symptoms or indicators.

B. Pain or Discomfort:

- It is normal and anticipated for cupping therapy to result in bruises and markings because the pressure and suction of the cups push blood and fluids to the skin's surface, where they form welts, blisters, and discolorations.

- Depending on the person's health, reaction, and recuperation, bruises and markings often go away in a few days or weeks and are neither hazardous or dangerous.

- Although they may be significant and indicate something, bruises and marks do not always indicate recovery. The quantity and quality of the blood and fluids, the kind and technique of cupping, the position and quantity of cups, the person's health and lifestyle, and the marks themselves may all affect the color, intensity, form, size, duration, and frequency of the markings.

Here are some pointers to reduce or control bleeding and scarring:

- Before and after cupping, use a moisturizing or calming lotion to nourish and shield the skin from dryness or irritation.

- After the session, apply a pressure bandage or a cold compress to the cupping area to prevent or treat swelling or inflammation, as well as to stop or lessen bleeding or bruising.

- To nourish and replenish the blood and tissues, as well

as to flush out the toxins and waste products generated by cupping, drink lots of water and eat a nutritious diet.

- Steer clear of the sun, heat, and cold since these factors might exacerbate skin discoloration or irritation.

- Steer clear of narcotics, alcohol, smoke, and extreme physical activity since they might impede the healing process or have unfavorable effects.

Several indications or symptoms that might point to a major issue or severe bruising include:

- The markings are painful, big, uneven, black, and persistent.

- They do not go away with time.

- Fever, rash, pus, infection, or the markings spread to other persons or places go along with the marks.

- Wet cupping is the cause of the markings, and the blood is extremely thick, black, or clotted, or it may contain contaminants or foreign objects.

- The patient has a history of medical issues, or they are on medication (blood thinners, thrombophilia, hemophilia) that affects blood clotting or circulation.

- Hematomas, hematuria, hemoptysis, or hematemesis are examples of abnormal or excessive bleeding or bruising in other areas of the body that the person experiences.

It is imperative that you cease cupping immediately and seek expert medical treatment as soon as possible if you encounter any of these symptoms or indicators.

C. Hygiene and Safety Concerns:

- Cupping therapy requires hygiene and safety since it includes touch and manipulation of the skin, blood, and fluids, all of which might carry or transmit germs, pathogens, or illnesses.

- Hygiene and safety can help to avoid or limit the danger of infection, cross-contamination, and problems, as well as provide a safe and effective cupping therapy experience.

- To preserve cleanliness and safety during cupping therapy, use sterile and disposable cups and equipment (e.g. needles, blades, cotton, or alcohol) and avoid sharing with others.

- Wearing gloves and masks, cleaning hands and arms before and after the session, and switching between persons or places.

- Cleaning and cleaning the cupping area before and after the session, as well as covering or treating any sores or punctures that occur.

- Properly disposing of garbage and materials, such as in a biohazard container or sealed bag, while according to local waste management standards or legislation.

- Checking and updating clients' medical histories and records, as well as screening them for any signs or symptoms of infection or sickness, such as fever, rash, or pus, before to each session.

- Reporting and documenting any problems or accidents that occur during or after the session, such as bleeding, infection, or an allergic response, and getting medical assistance as needed.

Signs or symptoms that may suggest inadequate hygiene, safety, or a major concern include:

- The cups or equipment are unclean, rusted, or broken, and may include traces of blood or fluids from prior users, individuals, or regions.

- The cupping practitioner or client does not use gloves or masks, nor do they wash their hands or arms before or after the session, or when moving between persons or regions.

- The cupping region is not washed or sterilized prior to or following the treatment, and any sores or punctures are left untreated.

- Waste or materials are not properly disposed of, such as in a conventional trash can or an open bag, and are left in the cupping area or the environment.

- The customers' medical histories or records are not verified or updated, and they are not evaluated for any indications or symptoms of illness or sickness before to the session.

- Incidents or accidents that occur during or after the session are not reported or recorded, and medical treatment is not sought when needed.

If you detect or experience any of these signs or symptoms, stop cupping right once and get expert medical help as soon as possible.

Emotional and Psychological Responses:

- Emotional and psychological responses to cupping therapy are feasible and natural, since cupping involves stimulation and manipulation of the body and mind, which may impact the individual's mood, emotion, and cognition.

- Emotional and psychological responses might be pleasant or negative, moderate or intense, depending on the individual's personality, temperament, and expectations, as well as the type and method of cupping used and the setting and surroundings of the session.

- Emotional and psychological responses can be positive or negative, fleeting or long-lasting, depending on the individual's coping and adaption skills, as well as the support and advice of the cupping practitioner and others.

Here are some strategies for dealing with emotional and psychological responses:

- Recognize and embrace your feelings and ideas without judging or suppressing them, since they are natural and genuine and may give valuable feedback and insight into your health and development.

- Express and convey your feelings and ideas, rather than hiding or isolating them, as they may aid in the release and relief of stress and tension, as well as helping the cupping practitioner and others better understand and assist you.

- Manage and manage your emotions and thoughts; do not allow them to overpower or rule you, since they can influence your behavior and outcome, as well as interfere with the cupping treatment process and aims.

- Seek and accept professional treatment and support without hesitation or refusal, as they may provide expert guidance and intervention, improving your emotional and psychological well-being and quality of life.

Some indications or symptoms that may suggest extreme emotional or psychological reactions or a major condition are:

- The feelings and ideas are extremely unpleasant, strong, or unreasonable, and they do not alter or better after the session, or even after a few hours or days.

- Physical or behavioral changes occur in conjunction with emotions and thoughts, such as changes in hunger, sleep, energy, or activity, as well as withdrawal, anger, or self-harm.

- Traumatic or stressful events or experiences, such as abuse, violence, or loss, can trigger feelings and thoughts, as can underlying mental health problems like depression, anxiety, or PTSD.

- The individual has a pre-existing mental health problem or is currently taking medicine that affects mood, emotion, or cognition, such as antidepressants, antianxiety, or antipsychotics.

- The individual is experiencing significant or persistent emotional or psychological discomfort or impairment, such as suicide ideation, panic attacks, or psychosis.

If you see any of these signs or symptoms, stop cupping right once and get expert medical help as soon as possible.

Advanced Troubleshooting:

Uncommon Reactions:

- Uncommon reactions are uncommon and unforeseen consequences or outcomes of cupping therapy; generally speaking, cupping is a safe and successful treatment that has no major negative effects.

- Depending on the patient's health, response, and recuperation as well as the kind and technique of cupping, the setting and context of the session, and other factors, uncommon reactions can range from moderate to severe and be either transient or permanent.

- By adhering to the sterile and disposable cups and equipment, donning gloves and masks, cleaning and disinfecting the cupping area, and properly disposing of the waste, as well as by reviewing and updating the clients' medical histories and records and screening them for any indications of illness or infection prior to the session, unusual reactions can be avoided or minimized.

Some tips to address uncommon reactions are:

- Identify and recognize unusual reactions; do not ignore or dismiss them, since they may indicate a serious or life-threatening condition or problem that necessitates prompt attention and care.

- Report and document any unusual reactions, rather than concealing or denying them, because they may help the cupping practitioner and others better understand and assist you, as well as prevent or lessen the recurrence or severity of the unusual reactions.

- Seek and get competent medical advice and treatment without delay or refusal, as they may provide you with expert diagnosis and management, enhance your health and function, and even save your life.

Some examples of uncommon reactions are:

- Allergic responses are hypersensitive or unfavorable immune system reactions to the cups, equipment, or substances used in cupping therapy, such as latex, metal, or alcohol, that can cause symptoms such as itching, rash, hives, swelling, or anaphylaxis.

- Medical crises are sudden or serious conditions or issues that can arise during or after cupping therapy, such as a heart attack, stroke, or seizure, and cause symptoms including chest discomfort, shortness of breath, dizziness, or loss of consciousness.

- Unique cases refer to unusual or extraordinary conditions or scenarios that may emerge during or after cupping therapy, such as pregnancy, lactation, or menstruation, and may result in symptoms or consequences such as contractions, bleeding, or infection.

If you have any of these unusual symptoms, you should discontinue cupping and seek expert medical attention as soon as possible.

Legal and ethical issues:

- Legal and ethical issues are essential and relevant components of cupping therapy since it involves touch and manipulation of the body and mind, which may affect the rights, duties, and relationships between the cupping practitioner and the client, as well as society and the law.

- Legal and ethical issues might be favorable or negative, simple or difficult, based on cultural and religious beliefs and norms, country and state legislation and laws, and the session's scenario and circumstances.

- Legal and ethical issues can be avoided or resolved by adhering to the legal and ethical standards and guidelines of cupping therapy, such as obtaining the cupping practitioner's qualification and certification, obtaining the client's consent and feedback, respecting the client's privacy and confidentiality, advertising and promoting the cupping therapy in a truthful and accurate manner, and communicating and cooperating with the cupping practitioner.

- To cope with legal and ethical difficulties, it's important to stay knowledgeable and aware of their potential impact on your rights, obligations, and relationships.

- Be honest and transparent about legal and ethical difficulties, and avoid dishonest or deceitful behavior, as they can harm your trust, reputation, and credibility, as well as produce legal or ethical problems or conflicts.

- Be polite and attentive of legal and ethical problems, and avoid being disrespectful or careless, since this may offend or injure your cupping practitioner or client, society, or the law, and may result in legal or ethical complaints or conflicts.

Some examples of legal and ethical issues are:

- Legal considerations: these are the laws and guidelines that control the cupping therapy profession and its practice. Examples include the cupping practitioner's registration and license, the scope and limitations of the cupping therapy, the client's and the practitioner's liability insurance, and the reporting and documentation of the cupping therapy sessions and results.

- Ethical guidelines, which are the values and principles that direct the conduct and behavior of the cupping practitioner and the client. These include the cupping practitioner's competence and integrity, the client's autonomy and dignity, the cupping therapy's beneficence and nonmaleficence, and the cupping therapy's justice and fairness.

- Complaints and disputes: These are arguments or conflicts that may occur between the client and the cupping practitioner, or between society and the law, because of moral or legal concerns, such as the client's discomfort or injury, the cupping practitioner's malpractice or negligence, the cupping therapy's deception or fraud, or the infringement or violation of someone else's rights.

We trust that this chapter has given you a thorough understanding of cupping therapy and has assisted you in resolving any queries or problems you may have or run into during cupping therapy sessions. It is highly recommended that you stay in constant contact with both your cupping practitioner and your client, sharing your thoughts and experiences on the treatment. By doing so, you will be able to increase the efficacy and quality of cupping therapy as well as the satisfaction and overall health of all involved. We also stress the significance of consulting a professional for guidance and support with any particular or severe issues you may experience or have while receiving cupping therapy. Doing so will protect your health and safety and help avoid or address any issues or consequences.

You've finished reading this book, which has taught you about Hijama cupping therapy, a traditional, all-natural method of healing that has been utilized for ages by many different civilizations. Hijama cupping therapy uses suction pressure to force blood toward the skin, clearing the surrounding tissues of pollutants and toxins. Numerous medical ailments, including varicose veins, migraines, back pain, and blood disorders, can be helped by it.

You have studied about the Hijama cupping therapy's background, significance, kinds, methods, safety measures, and outcomes in this book. Additionally, you now know how to wear a hijab securely and successfully by following the right procedures and maintaining good cleanliness. With the newfound information and abilities, you possess, you will be able to practice Hijama on both yourself and other people and reap the physical, psychological, and spiritual rewards of doing so.

I hope that this book has inspired you to appreciate the wisdom and the beauty of nature, which has given us this wonderful gift of Hijama. I sincerely hope you will keep researching and learning more about this age-old, holy healing practice, as well as spreading awareness of it to others who might find it useful. It is my wish that you will feel the happiness and tranquility that come with leading a balanced and healthful lifestyle.

Thank you for reading this book. I hope you enjoyed it and found it useful.

Made in the USA
Monee, IL
07 July 2026

56551578R00197